the consumer guide to
vitamins

How to choose Vitamins, Minerals
and Other Supplements

Angela Dowden and Grahame Lacey

PAN BOOKS

ADVICE TO READERS

If you suffer from any physical disorder or special conditions, please consult your doctor before taking vitamin or mineral supplements.

First published 1996 by Pan Books
an imprint of Macmillan Publishers Limited
25 Eccleston Place, London SW1W 9NF
and Basingstoke

Associated companies throughout the world

ISBN 0–330–34436–6

9 8 7 6 5 4 3 2 1

A CIP catalogue record for this book is available from the British Library

Photoset by Parker Typesetting Service, Leicester
Printed by Mackays of Chatham plc

CONTENTS

ACKNOWLEDGEMENTS

The authors would like to thank the following people:

Sarah Crossen, Judith Dainty and Mr Michael Lacey for their comments on the initial draft.

Dr Adrienne Mayes for her expert advice and constructive criticism.

This book is dedicated to the authors' families whose support made it possible:

To Cate, and sons Matthew and Sam.
To the Smiths, Tarplins and Dowdens, especially Christopher.

Introduction

The idea that a well-balanced diet is essential for a healthy body is nothing new. But despite the knowledge that proper nutrition can help us experience good health, few of us put this theory fully into practice. For instance, experts agree that we need at least 450g or 1lb (five good portions) of fruit and vegetables a day to provide vital vitamins and minerals. However, the vast majority of us eat less than half this amount.

As a nation we're a lot more interested in our health than ever before, but at the same time we've become more reliant on processed 'convenience' foods, which can lose essential nutrients along the way. Because the two concepts just don't fit together, we've turned to supplements to fill in the nutritional gaps – around one in three Britons now take supplements on a regular or semi-regular basis.

But we're not taking supplements just as insurance against bad diet. More and more people state they take supplements to deal with the effects of stress, to help protect against or combat disease, or to slow down the ageing process.

Whatever their reason for taking supplements, consumers have the right to expect well formulated and clearly labelled products that are safe to use. But more than anything, the public

want to know which supplements might be of benefit to them,
how to pick out the right supplements, and how much to take.

This book seeks to address these issues and others in a clear,
concise manner. It is designed with the consumer in mind, giving
honest, straightforward and unbiased advice on choosing and
using supplements. Use it as a guide to make quick and informed
decisions.

The Medicine's Act

Under the UK Medicine's Act, retailers are forbidden from
recommending any supplement as having a beneficial effect in
respect of the following conditions

- Tuberculosis
- Cancer
- Diabetes
- Epilepsy or fits
- Kidney disease
- Paralysis
- Cataract
- Locomotor ataxia
- Glaucoma
- Sexually transmitted disease

CHAPTER ONE

Food Supplements – The Fundamentals

The Basics

If you have ever tried to buy a supplement, you have probably been baffled by the choices available. So when choosing a supplement, what are the most important things to look out for?

1   Strength – **LOW or HIGH?**
    Most importantly, decide what you want it for:
    a   Prevention of vitamin and mineral deficiencies
        Everyday nutritional insurance
        Maintenance of health

    . . . a basic, *lower* potency product is probably sufficient.
    or:

    b   To help relieve an ailment
        To meet special nutritional needs
        To improve certain aspects of your health

    . . . you will need a *higher* potency supplement for your particular requirements.

2   Range of Nutrients

In multinutrient supplements, try to make sure you are getting a full range of nutrients. For example, a 'multivitamin & mineral' is not living up to its name if it only contains a dozen or so nutrients. Similarly, a full B complex formula should ideally contain all eight of the B group.

3   Ingredients

If you have special dietary restrictions, then check labels carefully to see which supplements meet your needs, e.g. yeast-free, dairy-free, gluten-free, vegetarian, vegan, and so on.

'No added sugar' on a label may simply mean that an artificial sweetener is used instead. (*See* Sweeteners: Cracking the Code, p. 9).

4   Price

If you are shopping on a tight budget, then the price of a product will be a major influence. However, looking for the lowest prices may not always mean that you are getting the best value. Some very cheap or bargain offer products, such as certain garlic, multivitamin, and cod liver oil products, contain so little of the active ingredients that they may give few health benefits.

So, to make the right choice for you, look at the:

STRENGTH → RANGE OF NUTRIENTS
→ INGREDIENTS → PRICE.

How to Read a Supplement Label

Most vitamin and mineral products are legally classified as food supplements, but some products, mainly herbal, are classed as licensed medicines.

As there are no EC or UK labelling laws relating specifically to food supplements, the Ministry of Agriculture, Fisheries and Food has agreed guidelines with the food supplement industry on how these products should be labelled. This means all supplement labels should at least provide certain pieces of information in a standard manner – making comparison of one product with another relatively easy.

For example, every label must carry an ingredients box which gives all the ingredients present in the supplement – including the non-active ones – in descending order by weight.

Separately, there will usually be a nutritional information panel, listing the vitamins and minerals in a prescribed order, with the percentage of the EC Recommended Daily Allowance (RDA) provided by the nutrients shown.

EC Recommended Daily Allowances – As Used On Supplement Labels

Vitamin	EC RDA	Mineral	EC RDA
Vitamin A	800µg	Calcium	800mg
Vitamin D	5µg	Phosphorus	800mg
Vitamin E	10mg	Iron	14mg
Vitamin C	60mg	Magnesium	300mg
Thiamin (vitamin B1)	1.4mg	Zinc	15mg
Riboflavin (vitamin B2)	1.6mg	Iodine	150µg
Niacin	18mg		
Vitamin B6	2mg		

Folacin (folic acid)	200μg
Vitamin B12	1μg
Biotin	0.15mg
Pantothenic acid	6mg

What Are RDAs?

Recommended Daily Allowances (RDAs) are not literal recommendations for vitamins and minerals at all! If they were, then an American consuming 300 microgrammes (μg) of folic acid a day would be deficient in this nutrient, whereas a European taking the same amount would be obtaining more than enough for health! (US RDA = 400μg, EC RDA = 200μg). RDAs, or their equivalent, are different from country to country because they are still largely a matter of scientific opinion. Even the EC RDAs listed in the table on pages 5–6 were a compromise between the individual figures of various European countries.

Because nutrient needs vary so much from person to person, RDAs can't be taken as recommendations for individuals. In fact the UK Department of Health has coined the phrase 'Reference Nutrient Intake' (RNI) instead of RDA, to remove the impression they are 'recommendations' for individuals.

What RDAs do provide is an estimate of the nutrient intake needed to cover the needs of the population as a whole. In fact the RDA is usually defined as the amount that covers the average needs of virtually all (97.5%) of the population.

RDA figures for vitamins and minerals are pitched at the level that is enough to prevent clinical deficiency of the nutrient, with an added margin of safety. What they do not reflect is the level needed for optimal health – a concept now being researched by many nutritional scientists. For example, 10mg (the EC RDA) of vitamin E is enough for vital functions such as normal growth and development, but around seven times this amount may be needed to protect against heart disease.

Making Sense Of A Sample Label

Evergreen's Vitamin B Complex
60 capsules

Directions: Swallow two capsules daily
with a meal **(4)**

Nutrition Information – Typical Values:

Per Two Capsules **(11)**		%RDA **(1)**
Thiamin (vitamin B1)	30 mg **(8)**	2143
Riboflavin (vitamin B2)	30 mg	1875
Niacin (vitamin B3)	50 mg	278
Vitamin B6	50 mg	2500
Folacin (folic acid)	300 µg	150
Vitamin B12	15 µg	1500
Biotin	0.15 mg	100
Pantothenic acid	30 mg	500
Choline	25 mg	*
Inositol	25 mg	*

*No RDA exists **(2)**

Ingredients: **(3)** Vitamin B6 (pyridoxine HC1),
niacin (as niacinamide) . . . etc.

Keep out of the reach of children **(9)**
Store tightly closed in a cool, dry place **(5)**

LOT: **(7)**   BEST BEFORE END : **(6)**

Evergreen's Vitamin Ltd, Any Street, Any Town, UK **(10)**

1 Indicates the percentage of the EC Recommended Daily Allowance provided by the nutrient (on supplements for adults and children over four years).

2 Some nutrients have not been designated an RDA.

3 All ingredients are listed in descending weight order. This includes nutrients and other ingredients used to formulate the supplement.

4 These are the manufacturer's recommended usage instructions.

5 Follow the storage instructions carefully. Supplements should generally be kept in a cool, dry place in the original container.

6 The product should be used before the 'Best Before' date to assure full potency.

7 All products must bear a lot or batch number for full traceability.

8 Milligrammes (mg) and microgrammes (μg) are the units of measurement for vitamins and minerals. A milligramme equals 1/1000 gramme, and a microgramme equals 1/1000 milligramme.

9 All supplements, particularly iron, should be kept out of the reach of children.

10 The manufacturer's, or distributor's, name and address are required to appear on the label.

11 Nutritional information is given per quantified amount of the supplement to be taken at any one time – in this case per two capsules.

Sweeteners: Cracking the Code

Some people feel that if you are taking a 'health' supplement, then the last thing you want to see in it is sugar or a sweetener. Sugar contains no micronutrients itself, and so, it is argued, has no place in a supplement.

A glance down many supplement labels reveals that often sugar, in one of its many guises, or a sweetener, has been added to the product. If a tablet or lozenge is designed to be sucked or chewed, then usually a sweetener is desirable, to make the supplement palatable.

But in some other vitamin and herbal supplements, sugars or sweeteners account for a large proportion of the tablet weight. Sugars may be undesirable for diabetics, those following anti-Candida diets and other groups. Some people may need, or want, to avoid artificial sweeteners.

No Added Sugar?

Crack the sugar code by using our list of sugars and sweeteners below. 'No added sugar' on a label may mean that other sweeteners are used instead.

Sugars include: sucrose (ordinary table sugar), glucose (also known as dextrose), lactose (milk sugar), fructose (fruit sugar), and maltose (malt sugar). Raw cane sugar, glucose syrup, corn syrup and honey are all sugars, too.

Maltodextrin, from corn (maize) starch, is a type of complex sugar which may sometimes be used in supplements.

Sorbitol, **mannitol** and **xylitol** are sugar alcohols. In foods and confectionery, sugar alcohols are often used as a sucrose substitute for diabetics, as they do not require insulin for their metabolism. However in supplements, they are more commonly used as bulking agents rather than sweeteners. They have the same or less sweetness than sugar, but are of little use in low calorie diets because their energy value is close to sucrose (sugar).

Saccharin is at least 250 times sweeter than sugar. It is not widely used in supplements but does appear in some. There has been concern about harmful effects on the bladder arising from high intakes of this artificial sweetener.

Aspartame (trade name Nutrasweet), is 200 times sweeter than sugar, so only tiny amounts are needed. It is made from the amino acids 1-aspartic acid and 1-phenylalanine, plus methyl alcohol; it is broken down in the body to its constituents. Those who suffer from the genetic disease PKU need to avoid aspartame.

Acesulphame K is another artificial sweetener, and is about 130 times as sweet as sucrose. It passes through the body unchanged.

Excipients

Excipients are the non-active (non-nutritional) ingredients found in a supplement. For example they are necessary for formulation purposes e.g. to help a tablet hold together, or as processing aids e.g. to improve the flow characteristics of a powder, or perhaps as a coating agent.

There are a number of excipients that can be used in supplements, in quantities as laid down by European legislation. All are deemed safe, but some are generally thought to be more 'natural' than others. Here are a list of the major ones that you may see in the ingredients list on labels:

Microcrystalline cellulose

Tabletting binder and disintegrant. It is made from the cellulose walls of plant fibres that have been fragmented into microscopic crystals.

Methyl cellulose, Hydroxypropyl methyl cellulose, Hydroxypropyl cellulose.

In supplements these are usually used as glazing agents, giving a smooth film coating on tablets. They may also be used as slow release agents. Despite their chemical sounding names, they are essentially of natural origin, being derived from vegetable cellulose.

Copovidone

A bulking agent prepared by chemical synthesis.

Polysorbate 80 (E433)

An emulsifier derived from the sugar alcohol, sorbitol.

Di-calcium phosphate

May be used as source of calcium in supplements, but also used as a binding and bulking agent.

Carnauba wax, Shellac, Beeswax.

These three may be used as a glazing agent in tablet coating. Shellac is a substance made from the resin produced by the lac insect, whilst carnauba wax is obtained from the surface of leaves of the Brazilian wax palm. Beeswax may also be used as a release agent, e.g. in capsule royal jelly formulations.

Lactose, Sorbitol, Xylitol.

Commonly used as bulking agents or to aid compression; they also have a sweetening effect.

Magnesium stearate, Stearic acid.

Fat-based lubricants that stop tablets sticking to the tablet press during compression. May be of animal or vegetable source.

Vegetable fat (hydrogenated vegetable oil)

Used as a lubricant or slow release aid in tablets. Levels in supplements are insignificant in terms of daily dietary intake.

Silicon dioxide (silica)
Magnesium silicate
Talc

Commonly used as a flow aid/anti-caking ingredient in supplements – they help powder move through machinery. Silicon dioxide is a naturally occurring rock-forming mineral (present in sand) that may also be listed in products as an active ingredient. Magnesium silicate is made from magnesium oxide and silicon dioxide. Talc is a naturally occurring source of magnesium silicate.

Maize starch
Modified starch
Croscarmellose sodium (carboxymethylcellulose)
> These are usually used as disintegrants – helping a supplement
> to dissolve in the gut after it is consumed.

Flavours

Some supplements may contain flavours. Those most commonly used are natural vanilla (or its chemically synthesised counterpart vanillin), cocoa (also gives a brown colour) and citrus oils.

Colours

Some supplements may also contain colours, such as titanium dioxide (a white surface colour prepared from the mineral ilmenite) and iron oxide (rust). Natural colours include annatto (a vegetable dye from the seed pods of the tropical annatto tree), curcumin (from turmeric), chlorophyll (green plant pigment), and anthocyanins (a range of natural plant pigments).

Riboflavin (vitamin B2), an active ingredient in many vitamin preparations, is also a naturally occurring yellow dye.

Supplement Presentations

Supplements can be presented in all sorts of different ways, including tablets, capsules, powders and as effervescent formulations.

Hard Gelatin Capsules

Hard gelatin capsules are from animal origin, and are made of two separate interlocking pieces. They are a convenient way of providing a unit dose of powdered supplement, and break down quickly in the gut. Occasionally hard gelatin capsules may also hold liquid based supplements.

Advantages: Hard gelatin capsules usually contain fewer excipients (non-active) ingredients than tablets. They are generally easier to swallow than equivalent tablet formulations and may also be pulled apart and the powder taken separately.

Disadvantages: Not suitable for vegetarians or vegans.

Note: There are now some two piece capsules available which are starch or seaweed-based, and not made from animal gelatin. However, they are not as yet widely available due to technical limitations and usually cost a little more. In time, they will probably become more common.

Soft Gelatin Capsules

Soft gelatin capsules are used to encapsulate unit dosages of liquid based supplements such as cod liver oil. They are made from a mixture of animal gelatin and glycerin (a by-product of the manufacture of fats and oils).

Advantages: Market research shows that people find soft gelatin capsules the most acceptable and easy to swallow supplement form.

Disadvantages: Not suitable for vegetarians or vegans.

Tablets

Tablets are one of the commonest supplement presentations. They are made by mixing together all the relevant powder ingredients and compressing these into a tablet using very high pressures.

Advantages: Many tablet formulations are suitable for vegetarians and vegans. Tablets are also relatively less expensive than comparable hard and soft gelatin capsules.

Disadvantages: Some people don't find tablets as easy to swallow as capsules.

Chewable Tablets

Chewable tablets are commonly used for children's formulations, and are also often used for calcium, multivitamin and vitamin C formulations.

Advantages: Pleasant to take and portable – you can take them without water. Good if you can't swallow tablets or capsules.

Disadvantages: Usually contain sugar or a sweetener, which may be unacceptable to some users.

Liquids

Some supplements are available in the more traditional liquid form, e.g. cod liver oil, iron, royal jelly, ginseng.

Advantages: Easily assimilated, and suitable for people who cannot swallow tablets and capsules. Liquids are also a good way of getting a high potency supplement without taking multiple doses.

Disadvantages: It may be difficult to control dosage unless a proper measuring spoon is used, and liquids in bottles are not very portable. High levels of sugars or sweeteners can sometimes be present.

Powders

Supplements may occasionally come as powders, usually to be mixed with fluids.

Advantages: Suitable for people who cannot swallow tablets or capsules.

Disadvantages: Not very convenient to take, and dosage is hard to control. Powders are difficult to protect from moisture, and there is a possible risk of contamination.

Effervescent Tablets

Effervescent tablets are a common way of providing vitamin C and other nutrients.

Advantages: Very pleasant way of taking the nutrient.

Disadvantages: Expensive; the tablets may also contain sweeteners, flavourings and other additives which some people may feel are unnecessary or undesirable.

Slow Release Preparations

Because water soluble B and C vitamins cannot be stored in the body, a sudden high influx may super-saturate the system leading to the loss of these nutrients via urine.

To prevent wastage of Vitamin C and the B complex, products containing high levels may therefore be presented in a slow release form (also known as sustained release, timed release or prolonged release). Slow release tablets are formulated to gradually release their nutrients for absorption over a period of around 6 hours. This is usually achieved through using a special tablet core which is resistant to the watery internals of the gut, and which slowly erodes through digestive processes.

Slow release tablets should be taken immediately after a main meal in order to slow their progression through the gut and to allow enough time for the nutrients to be released.

Where do Vitamins Come From?

Vitamin pills don't grow on trees, so are they as natural as they're made out to be?

Many health-conscious consumers would like to think the nutrients in their supplements come from wholesome foods such as oranges, wheat and milk, but in the vast majority of cases this is not so.

Even if your vitamin C supplement does contain rosehips, blackcurrants or acerola cherries, the chances are these are only supporting ingredients, and the vitamin C actually comes from a powdered ascorbic acid source – straight from the factory! But there's a good reason for this: if you try and extract a vitamin from food, it is often destroyed in the process.

Occasionally, multivitamins may supply nutrients from natural sources (labels will state this clearly), but the levels will always be low by supplement standards, and the product likely to be more expensive.

Synthetic Can Equal Natural

To most people, synthetic means unnatural, undesirable and something to be avoided. But in it's true sense, synthetic is none of these things – it simply means that something complex has been 'built' using simpler building blocks. Nature is full of synthetic materials: the vegetable material that we eat has been synthesised from nitrogen and minerals obtained from the soil; and from carbon dioxide and water using the sun's energy – a process known as photosynthesis.

The vitamins in our supplements may have been synthesised in a manufacturing plant, but most are identical to those found in food, and therefore accepted by our bodies as natural substances. Granted, food does contain other components which could facilitate the vitamin's uptake or action, but these may be often added to well formulated supplements anyway, e.g. bioflavonoids with vitamin C.

Vitamin E: The Exception To The Rule

Something that isn't recognised as natural by our bodies is artificial, not synthetic. And when vitamin E is manufactured it's the main exception to the rule that synthetic vitamins are natural. Natural vitamin E is 'd'-alpha tocopherol, but when vitamin E is synthesised, artificial 'dl'-alpha tocopherol is formed. Consequently, synthesised vitamin E is not as active, weight for weight, as the natural version derived from a food source such as soya oil or wheatgerm oil.

How Are Vitamins Made?

The precise details of how many vitamins are synthesised are close trade secrets. However, some are made using bacterial fermentation processes (in which the bacterium is cleverly 'employed' to make the vitamin), or via chemical reactions. For example, vitamin C is made from glucose via a series of steps that mimic closely what happens in the bodies of animals who can make this vitamin.

What About Minerals?

Minerals are inorganic substances and therefore cannot be manufactured. They are part of the earth's crust, and we obtain them in our diets either from plants that have assimilated minerals from the soil (e.g. calcium in spinach), or from eating the animals that have consumed the plants (e.g. iron in liver).

Supplements that supply good amounts of minerals are usually made using minerals that have ultimately come directly from the ground. To facilitate their absorption from supplements, these inorganic minerals may be bound to organic matter, e.g. yeast or amino acids (*see* Absorbing Minerals, p. 64).

Vitamin and Mineral Safety

An excess of any food, even water, can be dangerous. But what about supplements? How safe are they, and are there any dangers from taking them over long periods?

Despite numerous scare stories, it's virtually impossible to overdose on vitamin pills providing you follow the label directions carefully. You can even take several supplements together, as long as the total level of any particular nutrient doesn't reach an unsafe level.

What Is An Unsafe Level?

This is a bit like asking 'how long is a piece of string?', as it is down to individual make up. Just as some of us have blue eyes and others brown, some of us could happily tolerate 9000 μg (30,000 iu) vitamin A per day, whilst others might start to show liver abnormalities at just 3000 μg (10,000 iu).

However, in establishing safe upper limits of intake, we have to be responsible and err on the side of caution, so that the figure used is based on one that has never been reported to harm a healthy person.

The Council for Responsible Nutrition (CRN), represents reputable supplement manufacturers in the UK. It published its scientific summary of safe upper levels (*Essential Nutrients in Supplements*), also adopted by other European supplement associations, in 1995 (*see* table below). Few supplements intended for self selection breach these levels, or similar ones published by the Proprietary Association of Great Britain, who represent suppliers of supplements to pharmacy outlets.

If you're concerned you might be overdoing your vitamin or mineral intake, take a good look at your labels, add up what you are getting, and use the table as a guide to ensure your total intake from supplements is within the bounds of safety.

Upper Safe Levels of Supplement Intake

Nutrient	Upper Safe Level for Self-Supplementation** (per day)
Vitamin A	2300µg (7660 iu)
Vitamin D	10µg (400 iu)
Vitamin E	800mg (1200 iu)
Vitamin C	2000mg
Thiamin	100mg
Riboflavin	200mg
Nicotinic acid*	150mg
Niacinamide	450mg
Vitamin B6	200mg
Folic acid	400µg
Vitamin B12	500µg
Biotin	0.5mg
Pantothenic acid	500mg
Beta carotene	20mg
Calcium	1500mg
Phosphorus	1500mg
Iron	15mg
Magnesium	350mg
Zinc	15mg
Iodine	500µg
Manganese	15mg
Molybdenum	200µg
Selenium	200µg

Copper	5mg
Chromium	200µg

*Niacinamide (nicotinamide) and nicotinic acid are two versions of niacin (vitamin B3). Nicotinic acid is not as safe in large quantities as niacinamide. This table assumes that one or the other form is taken, not both (check ingredients list on label).

**Higher supplement levels may be taken under the advice of a qualified health practitioner.

Note: The upper safe level of supplement intake for any given nutrient is in no way related to its Recommended Daily Allowance (*see* How to Read a Label, p. 5). For example, vitamin B6 products containing at least 100 times the RDA are considered safe, whereas long term daily intakes of supplemental zinc may be undesirable at only a little above the RDA.

Vitamin A And Pregnancy

With all the bad press that has existed on vitamin A and pregnancy, you might be forgiven for forgetting it's a vital nutrient needed for the healthy development of the foetus! A link has been suggested between the incidence of birth defects and vitamin A daily intakes above 3300 µg (11,000 iu) in pregnancy; however, no cases of vitamin A-induced birth defects have been reported in Britain. Nevertheless, pregnant women are advised not to eat liver – an understandable precaution as it is not unusual to find 30,000 µg (100,000 iu) in just one 4oz portion.

The government also requests that supplements containing more than the EC RDA (800 microgrammes) of vitamin A should carry label advice telling pregnant women not to take the product except on the advice of a doctor or antenatal clinic. So if you are pregnant, you will be fine taking a supplement containing vitamin A, but keep it down to 800 microgrammes a day. Of course you'd have to vastly exceed this amount before you risked hurting your baby, so don't panic if you were taking more than 800 microgrammes before you realised you were pregnant!

A Hungarian study (1992) including data from 1700 women, showed that a supplement containing 1800 microgrammes of vitamin A did not pose a threat to the unborn child, and in fact, its use was associated with a reduction in the level of birth defects.

Note: Beta carotene is often labelled in terms of vitamin A, but the vitamin is entirely non-toxic and does not count towards your daily vitamin A total from a toxicity point of view.

Claims

Why don't vitamin labels tell you what the product does?

You may have wondered why vitamin and other supplement labels don't give a clear indication of their potential use. For example, you may be taking a B complex to help deal with the effects of stress, vitamin C to prevent colds, or garlic to help lower your cholesterol level. But this sort of information is regarded as a 'medicinal claim', which supplements are not allowed to make by law.

On the whole, this is a good idea, as it prevents abuses of vulnerable people, who could be offered false hopes by a supplement claiming to cure cancer, arthritis or some other disease. But on the other hand the regulations at present can be overly restrictive – for example a non-scheduled nutrient (one without a Recommended Daily Allowance) cannot be mentioned anywhere on the label other than in the ingredients list, in the nutrition information panel or as a descriptive part of the supplement name. This means that nothing can be said about the functions of selenium on the label of a selenium product!

Reputable supplement manufacturers are happy not to make

medicinal claims, and to always stress that a healthy diet and lifestyle is more important than taking supplements. But they would like to be able to explain the function of all nutrients on the product label, and to continue to make 'health maintenance' claims which could help in making an informed product choice – for example 'vitamin C helps to maintain a healthy immune system', 'garlic may help to maintain a healthy heart' and 'B vitamins are needed for a healthy nervous system'.

The main problem is that various UK government departments cannot agree on what information should be allowed on a supplement label – there's even more argument between individual European countries! However, such differences are being slowly tackled, and we should eventually have an EC directive on nutrition and other claims to cover both ordinary foods and food supplements.

CHAPTER TWO

Vitamin Supplements

Multivitamins

A 'multivitamin' will contain a range of vitamins and often, though not always, some minerals. Both vitamins and minerals are essential for the normal functioning of our body. Some products are very basic and include only small amounts of selected vitamins and minerals. Others are more comprehensive and include a wide range of useful nutrients.

What Do They Do?

Many people choose to take a daily multivitamin as a form of 'nutritional health insurance'. For example, if you are concerned that your normal diet does not contain the right balance of vitamins and minerals for your own needs. Or if you do not eat a very varied diet, and cannot change it easily.

Many refined and processed foods, 'instant' foods, and foods that have been stored for some time often suffer from a loss of nutrient value. In these situations, a multivitamin can make up for any possible shortfall in your diet (though it would be better to improve your diet first!).

A general multivitamin may also help to boost your body's defences against infections and other minor illnesses, especially in winter. One study showed that in a group of elderly people (over-65s), a regular multivitamin and mineral supplement improved the immune system and reduced the risk of infections (*Lancet*, 1992).

At certain times, e.g. during or after illness, or during periods of stress, we may have an extra need for nutrients over and above the supply normally available from our diet. A multivitamin can help to meet this extra need. Even a good, 'balanced diet' cannot always supply all the vitamins and minerals we require when we have special needs.

Many groups of people are known to have extra requirements for vitamins and minerals:

- Those on restricted diets, e.g. coeliacs, diabetics, vegans, food allergy sufferers, etc.
- People with poor appetites, e.g. the elderly, the infirm.
- People who don't eat a wide range of foods, e.g. faddy eaters.
- People convalescing from illness.
- Those with a weakened immune system (suffer from frequent colds, infections, etc.).
- People with digestive disorders.
- Menstruating women.
- Pregnant and breast-feeding women.
- Slimmers (reduced calorie intake leads to poorer nutrient levels).
- Faddy children.
- Smokers and drinkers (extra need of antioxidants, in particular).
- Athletes and very active people.

Choosing A Multivitamin Supplement

Multivitamins are usually bought as tablets or gelatin capsules. There is a bewildering assortment of strengths and combinations, so which one is going to be best for you?

Two examples of different multivitamin products are illustrated on the following pages. They show you some of the things to look out for when choosing your multivitamin.

Product A shows what a typical low-strength multivitamin may contain. Product B shows what a more comprehensive, medium-strength multivitamin may provide.

So, what's the difference between these two multivitamins?

Product A will look and taste nicer, and will probably be smaller and easier to swallow. It has most of the key vitamins – but note no folic acid, which is an important B vitamin – and just a few minerals. Most nutrients are present at the EC RDA level.

It also includes a number of additives, some of which may not agree with sensitive individuals.

This formula is ideal for someone shopping on a budget, or who is looking for the bare minimum needed to prevent possible deficiencies of the major nutrients.

Product B gives a wider range of vitamins and minerals, and many are at moderate or more meaningful strengths, above the EC RDA. It would provide a better level of nutritional health insurance, or would be more suitable for those with special needs, or recovering after illness, etc. It also has fewer tablet additives than Product A.

Although it may cost a little more than Product A, Product B may be a more effective multivitamin supplement for many people.

So, check your labels to see what you're getting in your multivitamin!

Product A

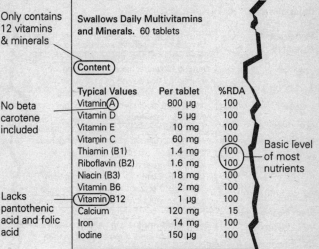

Only contains 12 vitamins & minerals

No beta carotene included

Lacks pantothenic acid and folic acid

Swallows Daily Multivitamins and Minerals. 60 tablets

Content

Typical Values	Per tablet	%RDA
Vitamin A	800 µg	100
Vitamin D	5 µg	100
Vitamin E	10 mg	100
Vitamin C	60 mg	100
Thiamin (B1)	1.4 mg	100
Riboflavin (B2)	1.6 mg	100
Niacin (B3)	18 mg	100
Vitamin B6	2 mg	100
Vitamin B12	1 µg	100
Calcium	120 mg	15
Iron	14 mg	100
Iodine	150 µg	100

Basic level of most nutrients

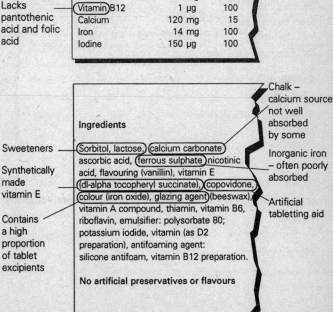

Sweeteners

Synthetically made vitamin E

Contains a high proportion of tablet excipients

Ingredients

Sorbitol, lactose, calcium carbonate ascorbic acid, ferrous sulphate, nicotinic acid, flavouring (vanillin), vitamin E (dl-alpha tocopheryl succinate), copovidone, colour (iron oxide), glazing agent (beeswax), vitamin A compound, thiamin, vitamin B6, riboflavin, emulsifier: polysorbate 80; potassium iodide, vitamin (as D2 preparation), antifoaming agent: silicone antifoam, vitamin B12 preparation.

No artificial preservatives or flavours

Chalk – calcium source not well absorbed by some

Inorganic iron – often poorly absorbed

Artificial tabletting aid

Product B

Most minerals
are in organic
form – easier
to absorb

Natural form
of vitamin E

Plant based
non-sugar
coating

Suitable for
people with
most allergies
or food
sensitivities.

Ingredients

Di-calcium phosphate, ascorbic acid,
magnesium citrate, zinc amino acid chelate,
ferrous fumarate, niacin (as niacinamide),
vitamin B6 (pyridoxine HCL), thiamin
mononitrate, riboflavin, beta carotene
preparation, pantothenic acid
(as calcium pantothenate), vitamin E
(as d-alpha tocopheryl acetate), magnesium
stearate, l-selenomethionine, hydrogenated
vegetable oil, potassium iodide, vitamin A
(as retinyl acetate preparation), folacin (as
folic acid), vitamin D, (as D3 preparation),
vitamin B12 preparation, biotin preparation,
glazing agent: hydroxypropylmethylcellulose.

No added sugar, no artificial preservatives,
colours or flavours. Free of yeast, wheat,
gluten and dairy products.

Capital "Multimax" Multivitamins and Minerals. 30 tablets

Includes 19 vitamins & minerals

(Content)

Typical Values	Per tablet	%RDA
Vitamin A	2800 µg	350
from: retinol	800 µg	*
beta carotene	2000 µg	*
Vitamin D	5 µg	100
Vitamin E	20 mg	200
Vitamin C	120 mg	200
Thiamin (B1)	10 mg	714
Riboflavin (B2)	12 mg	750
Niacin (B3)	45 mg	250
Vitamin B6	15 mg	750
Folacin (folic acid)	400 µg	200
Vitamin B12	10 µg	1000
Biotin	0.15 mg	100
Pantothenic acid (B5)	30 mg	500
Calcium	145 mg	18
Phosphorus	113 mg	14
Iron	14 mg	100
Magnesium	75 mg	25
Zinc	10 mg	66
Iodine	150 µg	100
Selenium	50 µg	*

*No RDA established.

Good levels of main antioxidants

Many nutrients are above the basic EC RDA

This means there is twice the EC RDA

All 8 B vitamins included

Buying Tips

Decide what you want a multivitamin for: are you after the basic minimum, with most vitamins at 100% EC RDA levels (such as Product A), or do you want one that offers a little more (such as Product B)?

If you are buying a particularly high potency ('mega dose') multivitamin, you may be better off with a slow release form, to help reduce potential wastage of water soluble vitamins (see Supplement Presentations, p. 16).

Multivitamin Mini-File

- *Can be used as a 'top-up' to protect your general health*
- *Useful if on a restricted diet*
- *Helpful at times of increased nutrient need*
- *Could help to improve your resistance to minor illnesses*
- *More effective if taken on a regular basis*
- *Differing product strengths to match your needs*

Children's Multivitamins

Most children's multivitamins are suitable for 3 to 12 year olds. They normally include sugars or sweeteners, sometimes as a high proportion of the chewable tablet or liquid – check labels to find out.

Some include only the basic, most essential vitamins A, C & D. Others include some iron (especially important for vegetarian children), but very few include many minerals. Minerals are as vital as vitamins for healthy growth and development.

As some children are sensitive to artificial additives, it is worth checking labels carefully to see what is included.

There have been a lot of claims and counter-claims concerning the role of vitamins and minerals in relation to a child's

IQ. Nutrition does play an important part in the development and functioning of the brain, but supplements won't enhance intelligence unless the child is poorly nourished to start with.

Vitamin A

Vitamin A (retinol) is a fat soluble vitamin that naturally occurs only in animal foods. The vitamin is measured in microgrammes (μg), but was formerly expressed in terms of international units (iu). For conversion purposes:

1 microgramme (μg) = 3.33 International Units (iu)

e.g. 800μg = 2664iu

What Does It Do?

Vitamin A is needed for healthy skin and eyes; it is a component of the eye pigment visual purple – essential for night-time vision. The vitamin is vital for the health of protective mucous surfaces in the respiratory, reproductive and gastrointestinal tracts, and also helps our immune defence system to function properly. Deficiency of vitamin A is rare in this country, but can lead to the skin becoming rough and hard, with blockage of the sebaceous (oil) glands.

Supplements of vitamin A are sometimes advocated in the skin conditions psoriasis and acne. However, high level vitamin A supplementation should always be under the control of a health practitioner.

How Much Do We Need?

The EC Recommended Daily Allowance (RDA) for vitamin A is 800 microgrammes, and this is sufficient for most people's needs. Beta carotene from vegetable sources can be converted by the body into vitamin A, but it is desirable to ensure an adequate intake of preformed vitamin A, so that beta carotene does not have to be diverted down this pathway, and can fulfil its antioxidant function.

Food Sources
Cod liver oil, halibut liver oil
Liver
Butter, eggs, cheese, milk
Herring, mackerel
Margarine is fortified with vitamin A

Choosing A Vitamin A Supplement
People most often take a vitamin A supplement to promote healthy skin, and to help build resistance to coughs, colds, etc.

Multivitamins and cod liver oil are the most popular vitamin A containing products, with a daily dose normally providing around the EC RDA (800µg) of vitamin A. Cod liver oil also provides vitamins D and sometimes E.

In multivitamins, the vitamin A is usually synthesised from vegetable sources, and therefore is suitable for vegetarians. Vitamin A can often be 'esterified' to make it more stable – hence you may see it listed in the ingredients list as 'palmitate', or 'acetate'. This makes no difference to the efficacy of the vitamin.

Safety
Vitamin A is stored in the liver, and can be toxic in excessive quantities. The maximum advisable intake of vitamin A from supplements is 2300 µg (7660iu) per day, but in actual practice, toxicity is not often seen until intake exceeds three times this.

Over-consumption of vitamin A is potentially most dangerous in pregnant women, as large doses can cause birth defects. Fortunately, there have been no such cases in the UK, but pregnant women are advised not to eat liver because of its very large vitamin A content. Additionally, supplements containing more than 800 microgrammes (μg) of preformed vitamin A (i.e. not as beta carotene) are required to carry warnings advising women not to take them except under medical guidance (*see also* Vitamin and Mineral Safety, p. 21).

Vitamin A Mini-File

- *Fat soluble vitamin*
- *Needed for healthy skin and mucous passages*
- *Helps build resistance to minor infections*
- *Necessary for night-time vision*
- *May help acne and psoriasis*
- *Excess should be avoided in pregnancy*
- *EC RDA = 800μg*

Beta Carotene

Beta carotene is one of a family of carotenoids that provide the pigmentation in plants. Hence vegetables and fruit rich in beta carotene tend to be vivid shades of orange, yellow and green (e.g. carrots, peppers, cantaloupe melon).

What Does It Do?

Beta carotene can be converted to vitamin A (retinol) in the body, with the conversion rate being:

1mg beta carotene = 167 microgrammes (μg) vitamin A

If the body is deficient in vitamin A, beta carotene will be diverted into its manufacture, and will carry out the functions of vitamin A in the body (*see* Vitamin A, p. 31); however beta carotene also acts in its own right as an antioxidant – helping to mop up excess highly reactive molecules called free radicals. Damage to cells by free radicals has been linked to ageing of the skin as well as to more serious diseases.

Many studies have shown that a low blood level of beta carotene predicts future risk of cancer – so a high dietary intake of beta carotene over the long term may be important in preventing this disease. However beta carotene cannot undo the damage of a lifetime's exposure to free radicals – the Helsinki ATBC (Alpha Tocopherol, Beta Carotene) Cancer Prevention Study published in 1994 did not find reduced incidence of lung cancer in heavy smokers who took supplements of the nutrient later in life.

Studies also show an association between low intake of beta carotene and cardiovascular disease. In one study (*Lancet*, 1993), involving 1500 men under the age of seventy, a strong link was made between high consumption of beta carotene (from carrots and green leafy vegetables), and reduced risk of heart attack. The highest incidence of heart attack was in smokers with low beta carotene levels.

How Much Do We Need?

There is not a Recommended Daily Allowance (RDA) for beta carotene intake, but the average daily intake is thought to be low at around 2mg–2.5mg per day. If we were to consume at least 5 servings of fruit and vegetables a day we would be consuming nearer 6mg beta carotene – an amount which is much more likely to have protective benefits. In fact some nutritionists recommend higher amounts of beta carotene (10mg–15mg) for optimal health.

Food Sources

Carrots, sweet potatoes, broccoli
Watercress, spinach, spring greens

Apricots, mangoes, cantaloupe melon
Red/yellow peppers, asparagus

Choosing A Beta Carotene Supplement

A beta carotene supplement may be useful for smokers (whilst they are giving up), people who do not eat fruit and vegetables regularly and people with a family history of heart disease or cancer. A supplement may also help protect the skin from sun damage (*see* below).

Beta carotene in supplements can either be synthesised, or extracted from microalgae which are naturally rich in this nutrient. The algae form is more expensive but some studies suggest it may be particularly well absorbed and utilised by the body. However, the synthesised form is a highly pure and reproducible material which has been used in the majority of clinical trials to date: there is plenty of evidence that the body can cope very well with this form.

Beta carotene is available singly in tablets, or soft/hard gelatin capsules, and may be part of a multivitamin or antioxidant formulation. A good antioxidant formulation will include 10mg–15mg beta carotene along with vitamin C, E, etc. Individual supplements are usually available in dosages up to 15mg. Sometimes beta carotene is labelled in terms of its vitamin A equivalency – in this case, a typical 15mg beta carotene supplement would be labelled as providing 2500µg (8325iu) vitamin A.

Beta Carotene And Skin

Photo-ageing of the skin – the primary cause of skin cancer – is brought about by the action of UV rays from the sun, promoting free radical activity in the skin.

If you are going on holiday where you will be exposed

to strong sun, pack some beta carotene capsules in your beach bag! Take beta carotene to help protect your skin for a month before you jet off into the sun, and for at least the duration of your holiday. But remember, beta carotene supplements will not protect from sunburn, so suntan lotion must be used.

Safety

Beta carotene supplements are safe in dosages up to around 20mg per day. More than 30mg may cause a yellow colouration of the skin, and may not be advisable over the long term. Excess beta carotene does not cause vitamin A toxicity, as the latter is not made from beta carotene if there are already sufficient supplies of the vitamin in the body. The vitamin A value of beta carotene – sometimes stated on supplement labels – does not therefore count towards your vitamin A supplement total, which is based solely on the preformed (retinol) vitamin. (*See* Vitamin and Mineral Safety, p. 20).

Beta Carotene Mini-File

- *Fat soluble antioxidant nutrient*
- *Mops up damaging 'free radicals'*
- *Helps protect skin against UV damage*
- *Low levels may be associated with cancer and heart disease*
- *Can be converted to vitamin A in the body*

B Complex Vitamins

The B complex comprises eight related watersoluble vitamins:

Thiamin (B1)
Riboflavin (B2)
Niacin (B3)
Vitamin B6 (pyridoxine)
Folic acid (folacin)
B12 (cobalamin)
Biotin
Pantothenic acid (B5)

B vitamins tend to occur as a group in the same types of foods. They are generally unstable to heat, and are easily leached into cooking water.

What Do They Do?

B complex vitamins are needed for the release of energy from food – B1, B2 and B3 are essential 'cogs' in the energy-releasing cycle which is at work in our cells every minute of the day and night. The B vitamins are also essential for a healthy nervous system – nerve tissue has very high energy requirements, and is particularly sensitive to any shortages of the Bs, such as in times of stress.

Collectively the B complex vitamins can play a part in maintaining the immune system; some Bs are particularly involved in supporting the body's defences. The B complex also helps to maintain a healthy digestive system, and is needed for healthy skin, hair and nails. The health of eyes and mouth can suffer if B vitamins are deficient in the diet; mouth ulcers have been related to low B vitamin status.

Research has also indicated that generous intakes of the B vitamins folic acid, vitamin B12 and vitamin B6, can benefit heart health. Low intakes of these vitamins causes high blood levels of a substance called homocysteine, which creates a risk factor for heart disease, strokes and other such disorders. (*New England Journal of Medicine*, 1995).

Individually, the B vitamins have important properties in their own right (*see* separate entries). For example folic acid is crucially involved in foetal development, and should be taken as a supplement prior to and during pregnancy.

How Much Do We Need?

The EC Recommended Daily Allowance (RDA) for each B vitamin varies from a fraction of a milligramme (vitamin B12) to nearly twenty milligrammes (niacin).

When we are under stress (emotional, mental or physical), we have a higher requirement for B vitamins; a high carbohydrate diet and alcohol can also increase our requirements of these important nutrients.

It is generally accepted that some groups have greater than normal requirements for certain B vitamins. These groups include:

Heavy drinkers
Contraceptive pill users
Pregnant women
People under lots of stress
The elderly

Food Sources

B complex vitamins tend to occur together in food. Different foods will be richer in some B vitamins than others. However, good general sources include:

Wholegrains and cereals
Liver, meat, poultry, fish
Milk, eggs
Leafy green vegetables
Brewer's yeast, yeast extract
Fortified breakfast cereals

B12 occurs mainly in animal foods, but is also found in yeast extracts and in some soya protein foods (TVP, tempeh, etc.)

Choline And Inositol

Although they are not true B vitamins, choline and inositol are important related factors which complement the B complex, and which are sometimes included in B complex supplements. Choline and inositol both function in the metabolism of fat in the liver, and choline also forms acetylcholine which transmits nerve impulses in the brain.

PABA (para-aminobenzoic acid), which is a part of the structure of folic acid, is also sometimes included in B complex supplements, but it has no major role to play in its own right. However, it is an ingredient in some sunscreen lotions, and high oral doses are occasionally advocated in the skin condition vitiligo.

Choosing A B Complex Supplement

B complexes are usually sold as tablets or capsules. Basic B complexes will provide the B vitamins at levels mostly around 100% the EC RDA – perhaps a bit more or less. If your diet isn't too good, your skin and hair need a boost, or you've got a bout of mouth ulcers, these types or formulation are adequate to make up deficiencies you may have in your diet. But some may not contain all eight B vitamins, so do count them on the label!

The more comprehensive formulations will contain all eight Bs, plus choline and inositol. They tend to be stronger, many of the Bs being present at 10 to 20 times (1000% to 2000%) the EC RDA, or more.

A sudden large influx of water soluble B vitamins into the body can result in their immediate loss via the urine, so some high strength products may have a 'slow release' action. This means they release their nutrients in a controlled manner over a longer period, to reduce the risk of wastage.

You may choose these higher strength formulations if you are particularly lacking energy, stressed or run down, and are in a high need category for B vitamins. Certain products, with 'stress protection' in mind, will include vitamin C along with the B vitamins, for added benefits. Look for these B plus C combinations if yours is a particularly demanding lifestyle or if stress has contributed to a lowering of your immune defences.

If you take a high dose single B vitamin supplement for a prolonged period, it may be best to take a modest B complex supplement as well, to prevent any possible imbalances or to improve effectiveness.

Brewer's Yeast

Brewer's yeast is sometimes taken as a natural source of the B vitamins. Compared on a weight for weight basis with ordinary foods, brewer's yeast is very nutrient-dense. However, compared with most purified B complex supplements, brewer's yeast is of weak potency; a typical daily intake of 6 x 300mg tablets often provides B vitamins at levels below the RDA. Consequently, brewer's yeast, though cheap, is not an efficient way of getting high supplemental levels of B vitamins.

Buying Tips

Check the strength of the B complex vitamin you are buying – does the strength match its intended use?

Make sure all eight of the B group vitamins are present – it's not a true B 'complex' if they are not!

If you are allergic to yeast in foods, or have suffered from thrush or a Candida albicans-type infection, you may need a 'yeast-free' B supplement. They are usually clearly marked as such on the label.

Safety

B vitamins have very low toxicity, and are normally entirely safe when taken as directed (*see* Vitamin and Mineral Safety, p. 20).

Note: Riboflavin (vitamin B2) is sometimes used as a food colouring – it may naturally turn your urine a deep yellow colour when taken in B complex supplements. This is an entirely harmless effect.

B Complex Mini-File

- *Eight individual B vitamins*
- *Needed for healthy nervous system*
- *Stress depletes the Bs*
- *May boost flagging energy levels*
- *Required for healthy skin, hair, digestive system*
- *Some people need B vitamins from a yeast-free source*

Pantothenic Acid (Vitamin B5)

Pantothenic acid/calcium pantothenate (vitamin B5) is a water soluble B complex vitamin. It is widely available in the diet ('panthos' in Greek means 'everywhere') and is sometimes known as the 'anti-stress' vitamin.

Pantothenic acid is fairly heat-resistant, and survives some cooking processes. However it is acid (e.g. vinegar), and alkali (e.g. bicarbonate) sensitive and is easily lost in cooking water.

What Does It Do?

Pantothenic acid is a constituent of coenzyme A, an important part of the cycle which releases energy from our food. It is also important for our immune system: it helps in the manufacture of antibodies which are needed to fight invading bacteria in our bodies.

The cortisone hormone – needed to help us cope with stress – is produced by the adrenal glands (sitting above the kidneys), and needs pantothenic acid for its formation. Cortisone has a mild anti-inflammatory effect, and some rheumatoid arthritis sufferers have noticed a reduction in the degree of pain and stiffness after taking extra pantothenic acid. In fact, arthritics are the most likely people to purchase this vitamin as an individual supplement.

Reports that high doses of pantothenic acid may reverse the greying of hair have not been supported in fact!

How Much Do We Need?

The EC Recommended Daily Allowance (RDA) is 6mg. The vitamin is not normally lacking in our diets, but alcoholics and those using long-term antibiotics may need extra. Stress may also mean we have an extra need for the vitamin.

Food Sources

Liver, chicken, beef
Brewer's yeast, yeast extract
Wheatgerm, oats, nuts, soya beans
Eggs and dairy products

Choosing A Pantothenic Acid Supplement

Pantothenic acid is usually included in B complex products, as well as in multivitamin formulations. As an individual supplement, it may be named calcium pantothenate or pantothenic acid, but the true potency relates to the latter. Common strengths of pantothenic acid are 100mg to around 500mg (check the 'Nutrition Information' panel on the label). The highest potencies may be in a 'slow release' form, which helps to minimise wastage of this water soluble vitamin.

Remember not to confuse calcium pantothenate with an ordinary calcium supplement – there is very little calcium in it, and the calcium is not readily absorbed.

Safety

Pantothenic acid is a very safe vitamin with no known toxic effects. The maximum daily amount normally supplied by supplements is 500mg.

Pantothenic Acid Mini-File

- *Needed for energy release from food*
- *Helps produce stress hormone cortisone*
- *Needed for antibody production*
- *Sometimes taken by arthritis sufferers*
- *EC RDA = 6mg*

Vitamin B6 (Pyridoxine)

Vitamin B6, also known as pyridoxine, is a member of the water-soluble B group. It occurs widely in the diet, but easily leaches out into water, and is also sensitive to alkalis (e.g. bicarbonate) and sunlight. B6 is sometimes called the 'anti-depression' vitamin.

What Does It Do?

Vitamin B6 is needed for the correct utilisation of proteins in the body, and also helps the nervous system in a number of ways. It is required for the production of serotonin, a brain chemical affecting mood, behaviour and sleep patterns.

Lower blood levels of vitamin B6 are sometimes found in women taking the contraceptive pill, and these low vitamin B6 levels may be related to mild depression. A supplement of the vitamin may have a calming and anti-depressive effect in such women.

Although not all trials have shown positive outcomes, one study of 630 women with premenstrual syndrome showed good results for many after supplementing with vitamin B6 on a regular basis. Carried out at St Thomas's Hospital, London (1988), the study showed improvements in PMS symptoms with daily intakes of vitamin B6 between 40mg and 200mg. Very few side effects were noted.

A lack of vitamin B6 may increase the risk of kidney stone formation in susceptible people. Taking B6 with the mineral magnesium may prevent kidney stones occurring.

Vitamin B6 has also been shown to be effective in preventing the onset of 'carpal tunnel syndrome' – inflammation of the nerve as it passes through the wrist. An effective dosage is 100mg–200mg daily for at least three months.

How Much Do We Need?

The EC Recommended Daily Allowance (RDA) for vitamin B6 is 2mg; more may be needed by people on high protein diets.

Food Sources

Wheatgerm, oats
Bananas
Chicken, white fish, liver
Nuts, potatoes, soya beans, milk

Choosing A Vitamin B6 Supplement

B6 is included in B complex and multivitamin products, but often at a low level, designed simply to make up for any inadequacies in intake of the vitamin from the diet.

If you want extra vitamin B6 for a specific purpose, choose a separate supplement providing 50mg or 100mg per day. Vitamin

B6 is often included at this sort of level in targeted premenstrual formulations, along with nutrients such as magnesium for added benefit.

Supplements containing 100mg or more of vitamin B6 may be 'slow-release' so there is less wastage of this water soluble nutrient.

Safety

Despite occasional claims that vitamin B6 can cause pins and needles at levels as low as 50mg, a thorough investigation of the safety data existing on the vitamin does not bear this out. For daily supplementation, a suggested maximum is 200mg.

Caution: High level vitamin B6 should not be taken with the Parkinson's disease medication levodopa, except under the advice of a medical practitioner.

Vitamin B6 Mini-File

- *Many women find B6 helpful for PMS*
- *Contraceptive pill/HRT can deplete B6*
- *Needed for protein metabolism*
- *Needed for healthy nervous system – 'anti-depressant' vitamin*
- *EC RDA = 2mg*

Vitamin B12

Vitamin B12 contains as part of its structure the mineral cobalt, and hence is also known as cobalamin. It is another member of the water soluble B complex, and is sometimes designated 'anti-pernicious factor' after its ability to prevent the condition pernicious anaemia.

What Does It Do?

Vitamin B12's function is closely interrelated with that of folic acid, and together the vitamins are involved in the production of new cells – particularly red blood cells. Vitamin B12 also helps in nervous function – it is needed for the health of the protective sheath around nerve fibres.

The absorption of vitamin B12 is dependent on the presence of a substance called intrinsic factor in gastric juices. Serious deficiency of vitamin B12 occurs in people who are not producing intrinsic factor, and results in pernicious anaemia. The disease may run in families, and can result from an abnormal immune response which destroys the mechanism for making intrinsic factor. Pernicious anaemia results in fewer, irregular red blood cells, but in the longer term, serious nervous symptoms result, which are irreversible if not treated with vitamin B12 in time.

According to research published in 1993 and carried out at Trinity College, Dublin, pregnant women may need to take a supplement of vitamin B12 as well as folic acid to reduce the risk of spina bifida babies. Vitamin B12 appears to be an independent risk factor: women with the lowest as compared with the highest intakes of this nutrient, were five times more likely to experience birth defects.

There have been claims that very large doses of vitamin B12 (up to 1mg or more) may reduce fatigue and improve mental function in the elderly. This type of usage should be under the advice of a health practitioner.

How Much Do We Need?

The EC Recommended Daily Allowance (RDA) for vitamin B12 is just 1 microgramme per day, although other authorities recommend 2 microgrammes per day, and requirements may be increased in pregnancy, lactation and in the elderly.

Higher intakes are perfectly safe, but do not appear to be necessary in normal healthy people.

Food Sources

Liver, meat, fish
Dairy products, eggs
Brewer's yeast, yeast extract
Fortified soya products
Fortified breakfast cereals

Choosing A Vitamin B12 Supplement

Pernicious anaemia due to an absence of intrinsic factor is a serious medical condition and must be treated with vitamin B12 injections – oral supplements are not effective.

However, vitamin B12 can sometimes be deficient in vegetarians and especially vegans, because animal foods are the main source of the vitamin. For these groups, a modest daily supplement is desirable. Similarly, elderly people or those with gastric problems may also require a supplement due to difficulties in absorption of the vitamin.

Vitamin B12 is a component of many multivitamin and B complex formulations, but can also be bought separately as tablets or capsules for those that require it. A typical, more than adequate dose is 10 microgrammes, but levels can vary widely.

Although vitamin B12 only occurs naturally in animal foods, the vitamin in supplements is usually prepared by a fermentation process. Tablet formulations are therefore normally suitable for vegetarians and vegans.

Spirulina, chlorella and other algae-type supplements also provide vitamin B12 in amounts above or around the RDA.

Safety

Vitamin B12 is a very safe vitamin, and there is no known toxic level. However, very few supplements supply more than 500 microgrammes.

Vitamin B12 Mini-File

- *Needed for manufacture of red blood cells*
- *Required for a healthy nervous system*
- *Requires intrinsic factor for absorption*
- *Deficiency results in pernicious anaemia and nerve damage*
- *EC RDA = 1µg*

Folic Acid

Folic acid, otherwise known as folacin or folate, is a B vitamin needed at a very fundamental level for the growth and reproduction of cells.

What Does It Do?

Red blood cells particularly need folic acid for their healthy development. A deficiency results in a specific type of anaemia (blood disorder) characterised by abnormally large red blood cells. The same type of anaemia is also produced by vitamin B12 deficiency.

Folic acid is also vital for healthy foetal development (see below), and some recent studies have shown it may help to keep the cells of the cervix healthy – low levels seem to be associated with cervical dysplasias, especially in women on the contraceptive pill.

How Much Do We Need?

The EC Recommended Daily Allowance (RDA) for folic acid is 200 microgrammes. Alcohol may reduce folic acid absorption from food, and blood folic acid levels may also be reduced by the contraceptive pill. The elderly sometimes have an extra need for this vitamin.

Food Sources

Leafy green vegetables
Wholemeal bread
Nuts
Liver
Soft grain white bread is fortified with folic acid, providing approximately 180µg per four slices.

Choosing A Folic Acid Supplement

Except in pregnancy, folic acid is not often taken as a supplement on its own. Folic acid commonly appears as an integral part of a B complex or multivitamin formulation, usually in levels around 50–200 microgrammes.

Most single folic acid supplements contain 400 microgrammes (though other strengths can be bought), and this is the strength to choose if you are planning to conceive, or are already pregnant. Certain folic acid supplements may also include other useful nutrients, such as vitamin B12, iron, calcium or fish oils. These are additionally recognised as being helpful during pregnancy, for the health of both foetus and mother.

Folic Acid And Pregnancy

Considerable scientific research over recent years has proved that folic acid helps prevent women giving birth to babies with 'neural tube' defects such as spina bifida.

These defects are due to failure of the vertebrae – bones of the backbone encompassing the spinal cord – to fuse during early foetal development.

Folic acid is essential for correct cell formation during the earlier stages of pregnancy. On the basis of the strong connection between folic acid and spina bifida, the Department of Health advises women planning a pregnancy to take a 400 microgramme folic acid supplement from prior to conception until the twelfth week of pregnancy. (In fact, it may be useful to take folic acid throughout pregnancy.)

Note: Women who have already given birth to one child with a neural tube defect need much larger amounts of folic acid if they are planning a further pregnancy. For this, medical advice must be sought.

Safety

Folic acid is in itself safe, but in rare cases, high levels may mask a deficiency of vitamin B12. Folic acid cures the noticeable anaemia symptoms of B12 shortage, but over a long period may allow the nervous damage of B12 deficiency to progress undetected.

Caution: Folic acid supplements should not be taken with epilepsy drugs, except on medical advice.

Folic Acid Mini-File

- *Needed for healthy cell growth and renewal*
- *Deficiency results in a type of anaemia*
- *Can help prevent certain birth defects*
- *Women need to take a supplement before they get pregnant*
- *EC RDA = 200 µg*

Other Single B Vitamin Supplements

Thiamin (vitamin B1): Alcoholics and the elderly are at highest risk of low thiamin levels. The vitamin may also be taken by holidaymakers, as it appears to deter biting insects in some people. Up to 100mg daily is the suggested level of intake for this purpose.

Riboflavin (vitamin B2): Deficiency of riboflavin can be associated with sore, cracked lips, mouth ulcers and tongue ailments; also with sore, bloodshot eyes and itchy eyelids. It is available as an individual supplement at dosages of around 50mg–100mg daily. Supplemental intakes frequently cause the urine to become a deep yellow/green colour – this is an entirely harmless phenomenon.

Niacin (vitamin B3): This vitamin is found in two forms, namely nicotinic acid and niacinamide (nicotinamide). Mega-doses of nicotinic acid can reduce high blood cholesterol levels, but restrictions on its sale mean that this use can only be under the guidance of a qualified practitioner. The maximum advisable supplemental intake of nicotinic acid is 150mg daily – higher levels can cause marked temporary flushing of the face and body. Niacinamide does not cause flushing, and is safer in higher amounts. However, it is of no use in lowering blood fats.

Biotin: A separate supplement of this B vitamin – needed for normal growth and body function – is sometimes taken by people with overgrowth of the fungal gut organism Candida albicans. It is thought to help prevent Candida albicans from developing into its more invasive form that can infect the bloodstream. A safe supplemental level of intake is up to 500 microgrammes daily.

Vitamin C

Vitamin C (ascorbic acid) is an important water soluble vitamin, popularly taken as a supplement to protect against colds. We need regular supplies of this vitamin, because the body cannot store it to any extent. Its major enemies are heat and water; storing fruit and vegetables will also lead to a decrease in their vitamin C content.

What Does It Do?

Vitamin C boosts our immune system, by strengthening the action of white blood cells that scavenge and destroy harmful bacteria and viruses (e.g. cold and flu viruses). The vitamin is also an important antioxidant, protecting the watery internal parts of cells from the ravages of excess free radicals (*see* Antioxidants, p. 64); it works in partnership with vitamin E which protects the fatty outer part of cells. Vitamin C can help to prevent cholesterol from becoming oxidised ('rancid') – a phenomenon now thought to be the precursor to the 'furring' of arteries; high intakes of vitamin C are also linked with lower rates of stomach cancer.

Vitamin C helps hold us together: it's needed for the manufacture of collagen – the intercellular cement of our skin, gums and tissues. Boosting vitamin C intake has been shown to speed up the healing process of wounds, as collagen helps to bind the broken skin cells together.

Vitamin C improves the absorption of iron from non-meat sources (such as bread or spinach), and so ensuring a good intake is useful if you are vegetarian, or prone to anaemia.

The vitamin has mild antihistamine properties, so some hayfever/allergy sufferers may find it helpful.

Furthermore, when we are under physical or mental stress, vitamin C is depleted from our adrenal glands: it's thought that the vitamin plays a regulatory role in the production of corticosteroid hormones such as cortisone which help us cope with the pressures of life. (*See also* Pantothenic Acid, p. 41).

How Much Do We Need?

The EC Recommended Daily Allowance (RDA) for vitamin C is 60mg per day, but smokers may need up to 80mg more just to keep their vitamin C status at the same level as non-smokers. Eminent researcher, Professor Anthony Diplock of Guy's and St Thomas's Hospitals, London, feels that the RDA for vitamin C is too low and that the full antioxidant benefits of the vitamin can only be gained with a minimum daily intake of 150mg–200mg.

For therapeutic effect, 1g or more of vitamin C may be needed daily, e.g. in colds. There may also be a dose-dependent effect: in heavy smokers, 200mg vitamin C only partially reduced genetic abnormalities in sperm, whereas 1000mg had much more effect.

Food Sources

Fresh fruit – especially citrus fruits, blackcurrants
Green vegetables – especially green peppers, Brussels sprouts
Potatoes (new ones contain more than old), other vegetables, including tomatoes
Fresh fruit juices – A glass of freshly squeezed orange juice (200ml) is one of the richest sources of vitamin C, containing around 70mg–80mg

Absorption

The total percentage of vitamin C absorbed is less from a high level than from a lower amount. For example, intakes of around 150mg per day are 80% to 95% absorbed, but a single 1500mg dose is only about 50% absorbed. In the play-off that exists between increasing dosage and decreasing absorption, an efficient high level supplement regimen is probably around

1000mg a day, either split into two 500mg tablets or taken as a single slow release tablet (*see* Supplement Presentations, p. 16).

Choosing A Vitamin C Supplement

Vitamin C supplements are widely available in dosages varying from less than 50mg to over 1000mg, and in chewable, powder and effervescent presentations as well as tablets and capsules. What level of vitamin C you choose depends on your reasons for taking the supplement: if you're simply boosting your dietary intake, levels near to the RDA will be satisfactory; however for more specific effects (e.g. reducing cold severity) you'll need to try much higher levels – probably around the 1000mg daily mark.

Some supplements state they contain rosehips, acerola etc., but these are almost always additional ingredients, and do not provide the bulk of vitamin C itself. In fact it makes no difference to the body whether the vitamin C it receives is synthesised, or from a natural source (*see* Where Do Vitamins Come From, p. 17).

Up to 500mg vitamin C, or more, can also be found in some antioxidant supplements, along with beta carotene, vitamin E, etc.

Buffered or low-acid varieties of vitamin C (usually calcium or magnesium ascorbate) are also available and may be more suitable for people with high stomach acidity, peptic ulcers, hiatus hernia, etc.

Buying Tips

Look out for vitamin C supplements that contain bioflavonoids – substances that occur naturally with vitamin C in foods (see page 56). They're not normally more expensive, and research shows bioflavonoids may enhance vitamin C absorption and augment its function in the body. But expensive 'patented' vitamin C formulations which claim better absorption through the use of vitamin C metabolites don't seem to be worth the extra money. A 1994 report in the Journal of the American Dietetic Association *found they weren't absorbed any better than plain ascorbic acid.*

Vitamin C And Colds

Vitamin C's role in the functioning of the immune system provides the basis for the theory that vitamin C supplements are preventive against the common cold. What does emerge from trials is that vitamin C can definitely reduce the severity and duration of a cold, even if it doesn't impact on the actual number we catch. The *Scandinavian Journal of Infectious Diseases* (1994) carried a review of 20 studies where at least 1000mg vitamin C was tested for its effects; although some of the studies found a link with fewer colds, all of them reported milder symptoms. These results may be of practical significance in terms of fewer sick days lost from work or school.

Safety

Up to several grammes of vitamin C (ascorbic acid) have been taken daily without reported side effects apart from transient diarrhoea. Based on extensive safety data, a sensible maximum daily intake is around 2000mg for most people. Higher levels are definitely not advisable in individuals with poor kidney function; however it is a myth that vitamin C causes kidney stones in healthy people. Similarly, reports that a person may suffer 'vitamin C withdrawal symptoms' after ceasing high level supplementation are completely unfounded.

Vitamin C Mini-File

- *Protective antioxidant*
- *Helps boost immune defences*
- *May reduce duration of colds*
- *Maintains healthy gums, teeth and skin*
- *Helps wound healing*
- *Helps iron uptake from vegetable sources*
- *EC RDA = 60mg . . . more needed by smokers*

Bioflavonoids

Bioflavonoids are a complex group of substances found in fruit and vegetables (particularly citrus fruit). Individual bioflavonoids include rutin, quercetin, hesperidin, etc.

In nature, bioflavonoids occur alongside vitamin C, and it has been shown that vitamin C is better absorbed in a citrus extract (i.e. when bioflavonoids are present), than alone. Hence, vitamin C supplements are sometimes formulated with bioflavonoids (check labels).

Bioflavonoids have also been demonstrated to have specific effects: these include a mild antihistamine and anti-inflammatory action, and a strengthening effect on the capillaries (tiny blood vessels).

In vitamin C products, bioflavonoids are usually present in relatively small amounts (up to around one tenth the vitamin C level) for the purpose of improving the vitamin's uptake.

Separate, stronger bioflavonoid products are also available. For example, rutin (from buckwheat) is popularly taken in tablet form. Typical users would include people with a tendency to bruise or bleed easily, hayfever sufferers or those with poor circulation or inflammatory conditions. As a guide, an effective intake of rutin would be around 120mg a day.

Vitamin D

Vitamin D is a fat soluble vitamin that naturally occurs in very high amounts in cod liver oil. Unlike other vitamins, vitamin D can actually be manufactured in our bodies – it is formed in the skin by the action of the sun on cholesterol. Since vitamin D is formed in one organ (the skin), yet acts on distant target organs (the gut and bones), it is technically a hormone.

What Does It Do?

Vitamin D is very important in regulating the metabolism of calcium and phosphorus, and is needed for strong, healthy bones. Vitamin D must first pass to the liver, and then via the kidneys before it is ready for action. If the calcium level of blood falls, the kidney is stimulated to secrete vitamin D hormone into the circulation, with the result that the gut absorption of calcium and phosphorus increases, and calcium is mobilised from bones into the circulation. This has the immediate effect of normalising blood calcium levels which must be kept constant for correct nerve and muscle function.

How Much Do We Need?

The EC RDA for vitamin D is 5 microgrammes (μg), although children and older people are liable to need more, whilst healthy adults who are outdoors quite a bit can manufacture sufficient to make a dietary source unnecessary. Dietary supplies of vitamin D are very few and far between, and the vitamin only occurs naturally in animal sources. Vegetarians – particularly those with dark skin, which doesn't synthesise vitamin D efficiently – may therefore need a supplement. Other people who may require extra vitamin D include the housebound elderly, lactating women and those whose religious beliefs require them to keep their skin covered.

Food Sources

Halibut liver oil, cod liver oil

Herrings, kippers

Canned sardines, tuna

Small amounts in full cream dairy products, eggs

Margarine is fortified with vitamin D

Which Number D?

Vitamin D2 (ergocalciferol) is a form of vitamin D that is manufactured using certain yeast organisms, and is suitable for vegetarians. However vitamin D2 preparations used in tablets may also contain animal gelatin.

Conversely, vitamin D3 (cholecalciferol) – the form of vitamin D naturally occurring in animal foods – may be synthesised in ways that make it suitable for vegetarians. For example, it is often manufactured from the cholesterol content of lanolin, obtained from the wool of living sheep.

The only real way to know if a supplement containing vitamin D is vegetarian is to read the small print on the label (or to ask the supplement supplier).

Choosing A Supplement

Young babies are often prescribed vitamin drops containing vitamin D because of its importance in early bone formation – talk to your doctor or health visitor about this. Vitamin formulations for older children also often contain vitamin D (usually 2.5μg–5μg per day).

A very popular way of taking vitamin D is as cod liver oil. A typical daily intake of cod liver oil (as capsules or liquid) provides 5μg–10μg along with vitamin A. You can also find vitamin D at a similar level in multivitamins.

Buying Tips

Look for vitamin D in calcium supplements. The vitamin helps with calcium absorption and should be a part of all formulations designed for bone health.

Rickets And Osteomalacia

Without vitamin D, people suffer major bone deformities such as rickets in children or osteomalacia in adults. In these diseases, there is poor calcification of bones, so that they are very weak. Full-blown osteomalacia is very uncommon in this country now, although mild cases quite commonly accompany osteoporosis in old age. Childhood rickets, although declining, is still too common, particularly in those of Asian origin. The disease can usually be prevented in all youngsters provided they obtain 10µg (400iu) vitamin D per day. This amount can be made in the cheeks of a European infant adequately exposed to the sun. However darker skin is not as efficient at making vitamin D, and in the winter, production falls considerably. The only secure way to ensure vitamin D intake in children is to give them a supplement.

Safety

Vitamin D is fat soluble and can be stored in the body, so excessive intakes can be harmful, initially causing loss of appetite, weight loss, nausea and depression. This type of effect could be expected from prolonged dietary intakes of 50µg (2000iu) per day. However to be safe, it's often recommended that the maximum daily intake from supplements should not exceed 10µg (400iu). This allows for a very generous intake of vitamin D from food – which most people don't achieve.

Vitamin D Mini-File

- *Can be made in the skin by action of sun*
- *Needed for strong bones*
- *Deficiency causes rickets or osteomalacia*
- *Young and old may need a supplement*
- *EC RDA = 5µg (200iu)*

Vitamin E

Vitamin E was discovered in 1922. Because it was found to be a factor needed for fertility in rats, the vitamin was heralded by some as an aphrodisiac – a reputation since proven to be a myth. However, vitamin E is very important for other aspects of our health, and has been the subject of a lot of recent scientific research.

What Does It Do?

Vitamin E is an important antioxidant nutrient – it helps protect fatty cell membranes from becoming oxidised ('rancid') through the action of highly reactive free radicals (*see* Antioxidants, p. 64). The vitamin is also needed for healthy red blood cells and proper functioning of the immune system.

Vitamin E used to be dubbed the 'vitamin in search of a deficiency disease'. It occurs in small amounts in a fairly wide range of foods, and it is rare that intakes are so low as to cause obvious deficiency symptoms. However, research over more recent years has shown that higher than normal dietary intakes of vitamin E may be associated with a protective effect against certain diseases associated with ageing – particularly cancer and heart disease (*see* pages 63, 67).

Vitamin E may be used to help improve blood circulation, and intakes of 300mg–400mg (450iu–600iu) have been found to improve symptoms of intermittent claudication (pain in the legs whilst walking, due to poor blood flow). Additionally some women find it useful in premenstrual syndrome, or in the hot flushes of the menopause, at levels of around 268mg–400mg (400iu–600iu) daily.

Vitamin E is also commonly used as a supplement to improve dry skin. Although there is no definite basis for its use in skin care, anecdotal reports do indicate it may be of benefit. Vitamin E is a constituent of many beauty creams that are applied to the face.

How Much Do We Need?

The EC Recommended Daily Allowance (RDA) for vitamin E is 10mg, while the Nutritional and Dietary Survey of British Adults (HMSO, 1990) found that the average daily intake of vitamin E was 11.7mg in men and 8.6mg in women. Our requirements vary according to our intake of polyunsaturated fats. These fats – found mostly in vegetable oils, nuts, seeds and oily fish – are thought to be more 'healthy' than the saturated kind. However they easily become oxidised ('rancid') in the body, and extra vitamin E is needed to protect against this.

Over recent years, research has indicated that an intake of vitamin E in excess of the RDA may be required for optimum nutritional benefit. For example 50mg–80mg vitamin E daily is associated with a higher antioxidant (protective) action in the body than the basic RDA level.

Food Sources

Wheatgerm oil
Sunflower seed oil, sunflower seeds
Hazelnuts, almonds, peanuts
Muesli
Spinach

Natural Versus Synthetic Vitamin E

Vitamin E is the only vitamin that is less active, weight for weight, when it is synthetically made. Manufactured vitamin E is known as dl-alpha tocopherol and is a mixture of eight compounds; vitamin E derived from a natural source (normally soya oil), is a single entity called d-alpha tocopherol, and possesses a higher biological activity.

Whichever source of vitamin E is used in supplements, the quantity (in milligrammes) on the label should always refer to d-alpha tocopherol equivalent; so 10mg of vitamin E stated on a label is equally active whether it comes from a natural or synthetic source. However, some users prefer to have natural source vitamin E. The synthetic variety is manufactured from by-products of the petroleum refining industry.

Choosing A Supplement

Individual supplements of vitamin E are usually available as oil based soft gelatin capsules – the oil (usually soya or wheatgerm) aids absorption of this fat soluble vitamin. Dosages offered are usually between 67mg (100iu) and 400mg (600iu) per day, a potency consistent with research indicating a potenially protective effect of vitamin E against disease. Capsules containing up to 670mg (1000iu) may also be available, usually for use with the advice of a practitioner.

Some vitamin E supplements may be offered in 'dry' tablet form – this form is useful for vegetarians and vegans, or for people who cannot absorb fat properly.

Vitamin E is usually also present in multivitamins – a level of 10mg–50mg being typical. This sort of potency is useful for people who do not eat proper balanced meals, and who consequently could be missing out on even basic intakes of vitamin E. Specific antioxidant formulations also provide vitamin E. A good antioxidant supplement should provide at least 67mg (100iu) per day.

In the ingredients list of some supplements, you may see vitamin E listed as an 'acetate' or 'succinate' form. All this means is that the vitamin has been made more stable for use in the particular formulation concerned.

Wheatgerm oil is a naturally rich food source of vitamin E, and is sometimes sold as an individual supplement, either as a liquid or in capsules. However it does not compare in strength with pure vitamin E products, with 10mg per capsule being typical.

Vitamin E And Heart Attacks

When it comes to heart attacks, vitamin E seems to show unique promise as a preventative agent. In two large US studies, significantly reduced heart attack risks were found in users of vitamin E supplements above 100iu (67mg) in strength (*New England Journal of Medicine*, 1993). Moreover, results from a World Health Organisation trial indicated that vitamin E status is an even more important predictor of heart disease than blood pressure or blood cholesterol.

Safety

Vitamin E, although a fat soluble vitamin, is very safe, and up to 800mg (1200iu) as a daily supplement is considered harmless. More may potentiate the effect of blood thinning drugs (e.g. warfarin), or cause occasional gastro-intestinal disturbance.

Vitamin E Mini-File

- *Fat soluble antioxidant vitamin*
- *May help improve condition of dry skin*
- *Helpful in maintaining a healthy circulation*
- *May be useful in PMS*
- *Could help protect against heart disease*

- *EC RDA = 10mg . . . more may be needed for long-term health protection*

Antioxidants

'Antioxidants' have become the nutritional buzzword of recent years, as more and more evidence shows how these protective nutrients can help to keep us healthy. The main antioxidant nutrients are beta carotene (the precursor to vitamin A found in vegetables), vitamin C, vitamin E and the mineral selenium.

What Do They Do?

Antioxidants help protect our cells from the environment in which we live. Just as butter goes rancid and iron nails rust when exposed to the oxygen in air, we too undergo a process of oxidation that may in the long run contribute to the several major diseases associated with ageing – including cancer, cardiovascular disease, rheumatoid arthritis and cataracts. Wrinkles and brown 'age spots' are also thought to be the result of oxidation.

Bringing about this oxidation are 'free radicals' – unstable and extremely reactive molecules which can cause damage to body cells and tissues in their attempt to become balanced. Free radicals are thought to be linked to cancerous changes in the genetic material of our cells. They may oxidise cholesterol, making it 'sticky' and more apt to stick to artery walls – a contributory factor in heart disease. Free radicals are also thought to play a role in conditions such as rheumatoid arthritis, maybe through 'attacking' the joints.

Free radicals are actually a natural by-product of the process whereby oxygen is combined with our food to produce energy. They are essential in controlled quantities for the vital function of destroying harmful bacteria. But in larger quantities, or if our intake of antioxidant nutrients is inadequate, free radicals can turn from friend to foe.

Excess free radicals arise mostly from environmental sources, including smoking, air pollution, X-rays and UV rays from the sun. However stress can increase the body's free radical load, as adrenalin forms free radicals when it is broken down after use. An excessive intake of polyunsaturated fats can also promote free radical action internally.

How Much Do We Need?

The EC Recommended Daily Allowances (RDAs) for the anti-oxidant vitamins C and E are 60mg and 10mg respectively. But some experts think that intakes to help prevent free radical related disease should be much higher than this: Professor Anthony Diplock of Guy's and St Thomas's Hospital, London, has suggested 100mg–150mg for vitamin C and 50mg–80mg for vitamin E. Whilst there is no RDA for beta carotene, it is thought that 10mg–15mg could be optimal, which is way above the 2mg–2.5mg average daily intake of British people. Selenium may also be needed in higher levels than normally found in our diets, if it is to act optimally as an antioxidant, e.g. keeping blood fats from becoming 'rancid'.

Food Sources

Beta carotene: Brightly coloured fruit and vegetables
Vitamin E: Nuts, grains, seeds, vegetable oils, especially wheat-germ oil
Vitamin C: Citrus fruits, green peppers, blackcurrants, potatoes
Selenium: Grains, fish, meat

Choosing An Antioxidant Supplement

You may choose an antioxidant supplement if you smoke (although a supplement cannot undo the damage of tobacco), if you are working or living in a polluted area, have a high exposure to X-rays, are highly stressed, or starting to notice the signs of ageing in your skin. An antioxidant supplement cannot substitute for a poor diet, but many people do take antioxidants if their busy lifestyles mean they can't be sure of eating at least five portions of fruit and vegetables daily (as recommended by the World Health Organisation).

Many multinutrient products are marketed as antioxidant supplements even though they only contain relatively small amounts of the antioxidant nutrients. A good antioxidant supplement should provide 150mg or more of vitamin C, 100iu (67mg) or more of vitamin E, 10mg–15mg beta carotene and 50–200 microgrammes (μg) selenium daily. More complete antioxidant supplements also contain zinc (5mg–15mg), and some also provide other nutrients involved in the body's antioxidant defence systems (e.g. copper, manganese and the amino acid 1-cysteine).

Certain antioxidant formulations may be based primarily on selenium (providing around 100μg–200μg per day), plus supporting nutrients such as zinc, vitamin E and vitamin C. These tend to be especially useful for people taking antioxidants to help with maintaining mobile joints (*see* Selenium, p. 86).

Some herbs have an antioxidant action (e.g. ginkgo biloba), and may also be included in antioxidant formulations. However, antioxidant herbs may not be present in effective quantities in multinutrient formulations, and they are usually better taken in separate herbal formulations at higher levels.

Similarly, coenzyme Q10 is also an antioxidant, but it has other functions, and is better taken separately to ensure an effective level (*see* Coenzyme Q10, p. 111).

Buying Tips

Look for formulations that contain antioxidant minerals (e.g. selenium and zinc) as well as antioxidant vitamins (vitamins C, E and beta carotene).

Antioxidants And Cancer Prevention

There have been around 200 studies of the relationship linking intake of antioxidant-rich fruit and vegetables and cancer. The overwhelming majority of these studies showed a protective effect of fruit and vegetables, with low dietary intakes carrying double the cancer risk of high intakes. Most people don't eat the recommended five servings a day of fruit and vegetables – so can antioxidants in a supplement form also provide cancer protective benefits? The answer for this is less clear, but one trial in which vitamin E, beta carotene and selenium supplements were given to a poorly nourished population in Linxian, China, did show benefits. In this population, which has the highest rate of digestive tract cancers anywhere in the world, the supplement reduced total cancer deaths by 13%, stomach cancer deaths by 21% and overall mortality by 9%.

Safety

Antioxidant supplements are safe provided they are used as directed. For more details on safety of the individual antioxidant vitamins and minerals, see the individual entries for these nutrients.

Antioxidants Mini-File

- *Vitamins C, E, beta carotene and selenium*
- *Protect cells from excess 'free radicals'*
- *Work against the effects of pollution*
- *May slow down ageing of skin*
- *May help prevent degenerative diseases*
- *Smokers need extra*

CHAPTER THREE

Mineral Supplements

Absorbing Minerals

Minerals – many of which are metals – are not found by themselves in food or supplements. In fact, most minerals naturally exist as mineral salts, e.g. iron oxide – the major constituent of iron ore. It is these compounds – known as salts – that are used as mineral sources in many supplements.

Mineral salts can be inorganic (e.g. chlorides, sulphates, oxides, carbonates), or organic (e.g. fumerates, gluconates, citrates, lactates). On the whole, minerals provided as organic salts – which contain a chain of carbon atoms – are better absorbed and/or tolerated by the body, although there may be exceptions for individual minerals.

Providing the mineral salt is soluble, the free mineral will be released on reaching the gut, and may then be absorbed. However, certain dietary components (e.g. phytic acid found in high fibre foods) may 'latch on' to the mineral, blocking its absorption.

Chelated Minerals

Absorption of minerals may be improved when a special bond, known as a chelate, is formed between the mineral and an organic component – usually an amino acid (protein building block). Instead of releasing the free mineral in the gut, the mineral and amino acid stay together and are absorbed as one entity. Hence, the mineral is not susceptible to being 'snatched' by phytic acid or other dietary components. As well as amino acid chelates, certain specific types of mineral chelate are sometimes used in supplements, e.g. zinc picolinate or seleno-methionine.

'Yeast-bound' minerals are also well absorbed. These are produced through cultivating the yeast organism in a mineral enriched environment, so that the mineral becomes incorporated within the yeast cell.

Calcium

Calcium is the most abundant mineral in the body, comprising over 1% of our total body weight. Of this 99% can be found in our teeth and bones, and the remaining 1% is found in soft tissues, including nerves, muscles and blood.

What Does It Do?

Calcium helps form the strong structural matrix of bones and teeth, but the levels in the body are not static: the bones act as a reservoir for calcium, and the mineral constantly moves in and out of this tissue. A constant blood calcium concentration is vital for health, so the bones release calcium if blood levels fall too low, or take it up if blood levels rise too high. The controlling mechanism for blood calcium levels involves special hormones and especially vitamin D, which improves calcium absorption from our food.

Insufficient calcium over a lifetime can lead to osteoporosis (brittle bone disease), particularly in post-menopausal women. Calcium deficiency, usually also combined with vitamin D deficiency, causes rickets in children, or osteomalacia (bone softening) in adults (*see* Vitamin D, p. 59).

Calcium is also needed for correct muscle contraction, including the heart muscle, and it works closely with the mineral magnesium in this regard. The mineral is also required for blood clotting.

How Much Do We Need?

In adults, around 500mg of calcium is excreted daily (mainly in the urine), and so we must get at least this amount in the diet simply to prevent a net loss from the body. The EC Recommended Daily Allowance (RDA) for calcium is 800mg; some groups, including teenagers and breast-feeding mums, need more.

Food Sources

Milk, cheese, yoghurt, cottage cheese, etc.
Sardines (tinned), eggs, tofu, fortified soya milk
Nuts (almonds, brazils – richest), sunflower and sesame seeds
Spinach, seaweeds, dried figs
Bread (calcium is added to white flour by law)

Dairy products are by far the best sources of calcium. A pint (568ml) of semi-skimmed milk provides 700mg of calcium, and a pot of plain, low fat yoghurt (150g) provides 285mg of calcium. Allergies to dairy products are relatively common though.

An Old Wives' Tale?

Drinking a mug of warm milk (rich in calcium) before bedtime to help you sleep better may not be such an old wives' tale after all! Calcium plays a role in nerve transmission and can help reduce irritability and mild hypertension. Insomnia is one possible sign of calcium deficiency.

Choosing A Calcium Supplement

Vitamin D is important for the absorption of calcium, so it makes sense for it to be included in calcium supplements. Many calcium products include some vitamin D, but some do not: read the label to find out.

An alternative is to take a multivitamin tablet, or cod liver oil (capsule or liquid) – both contain vitamin D – along with your calcium supplement.

Magnesium's functions also interlink with those of calcium, and many formulations aimed at general 'bone maintenance' include the two together. A lot of importance is attached to the relative amounts of calcium to magnesium in a supplement; but there is really nothing magical about the ratio of these two minerals! However, if a product does offer both, look for at least half as much magnesium as there is calcium; this falls in line with the relative requirements of the two minerals, and their amounts in body.

Zinc, manganese and copper are also essential minerals for bone synthesis, and may be included in calcium supplements. Similarly boron may play a part in maintaining bone, and is sometimes present in formulations for menopausal women.

If there are lots of 'extras' added (e.g. magnesium, zinc, etc.) there is less space for the calcium itself! If you are seriously concerned with getting very significant amounts of calcium (more than 800mg) from a supplement on a daily basis, you need to concentrate on a singular calcium supplement that can pack in the dosage because its formulation is not cluttered with other factors (although vitamin D is important).

You also need to think about how well a calcium supplement is going to be absorbed. The best absorbed forms of calcium are organic forms (as opposed to inorganic), e.g. calcium citrate, calcium gluconate, calcium lactate, amino acid chelated calcium and such like.

Inorganic calcium carbonate (chalk), is less bulky than other forms of calcium, providing more of the mineral in a smaller tablet. However, it may not deliver the calcium it promises, as it is insoluble, and as such, not well absorbed – especially in those with poor digestion. The same applies to di-calcium phosphate (calcium diphosphate), another calcium source commonly used in supplements. (*Note:* Dolomite – which comes from rock – is a cheap, naturally-occurring source of calcium and magnesium carbonates.)

Buying Tips

Check vitamin D is supplied in the product.

Decide how much calcium you need, and choose your product accordingly.

Check the calcium is in an organic easy-to-absorb form. Inorganic forms, e.g. calcium carbonate, calcium oxide and di-calcium phosphate, tend to be less well absorbed.

Calcium And Osteoporosis

After about the age of 35, bone tissue begins to lose more calcium than it can replace, and men and women will lose about 0.4% of their bone mass each year. This rate of bone loss is even greater (1%–2%) in women during and after the menopause. Why?

During the menopause, or 'change of life', a woman's oestrogen levels drop. Oestrogen protects against bone thinning in younger life, and as it declines, so does the calcium content of our bones. Osteoporosis may develop as the bones weaken and become more porous. In osteoporosis, the skeletal structure shrinks and causes the spine to curve. There may be spontaneous fractures, and a greater risk of bone fractures from falls.

Hormone replacement therapy (HRT) replaces the

lost oestrogen and aims to prevent calcium losses, but it doesn't suit everyone. A number of studies have shown hat supplementing the diet with around 1000mg calcium plus vitamin D can prove beneficial in reducing the risk of bone injury, by slowing down the rate of calcium loss.

The National Osteoporosis Society recommends a higher calcium intake for the nation in order to help prevent this crippling disease: 800mg for children aged 7–12 years; 1000mg for teenagers, adult men, and women on HRT; 1200mg for pregnant and breast-feeding mothers; 1500mg for pregnant teenagers and men and women over 45.

Weight-bearing exercise is also important for maintaining bone strength.

Safety

Up to 1500mg a day calcium as a supplement is thought to be safe, with any excess being easily excreted. Accumulations occur, e.g. kidney stones, only when the normal control mechanisms are no longer functioning. Certain diuretic drugs are 'calcium sparing', and increase the blood calcium level: follow your doctor's advice.

Calcium Mini-File
- Needed for strong teeth and bones
- Important for nerve and muscle function
- Vitamin D required for absorption
- Helps prevent osteoporosis
- Good calcium levels most important during our growth years
- If you don't sleep well, extra calcium may help
- EC RDA = 800mg . . . but more may be advisable

Iron

Iron is a vital trace mineral, needed only in small dietary amounts. The chemical symbol for iron is 'Fe', and on food and supplement labels, iron is often listed as a 'ferrous' compound, such as ferrous sulphate.

What Does It Do?

Iron is needed to make haemoglobin, the red pigment of blood. Haemoglobin is contained within red blood cells and transports oxygen around the body, from the lungs to the tissues, via the bloodstream. Insufficient iron to meet the body's needs can lead to iron deficiency anaemia. The symptoms are fatigue, light-headedness, pale skin and weakness.

Iron is also found in the protein myoglobin, the red pigment of muscles, and in certain cell enzymes. The remainder of the body's iron is stored in the liver, spleen and bone marrow. Iron stores may be up to 1g in men, but only about half this amount in women. Some women have no iron stores at all.

During pregnancy, there is an increase in iron absorption in an attempt to meet the needs of the growing baby with its own blood supply. However women who begin pregnancy with low iron stores may need iron supplements.

Recent evidence from the Ministry of Agriculture, Fisheries and Food, and the Department of Health, indicates that there is a high prevalence of iron deficiency in pre-school children. One- to three-year-olds should be consuming 6.9mg of iron daily – but over a quarter are getting less than this. Low iron intakes in this age group may result from an inadequate intake of meat, coupled with too many 'junk food' snacks.

Iron deficiency can occur after surgical blood loss, or if there is poor iron absorption from the diet, such as in coeliac's disease (where there is an allergy to the gluten in cereals). Vegetarians too are at risk of iron deficiency, as their diets only provide poorly absorbed iron.

How Much Do We Need?

The EC Recommended Daily Allowance (RDA) for iron is 14mg – based on an absorption of 10% from a mixed diet. It is acknowledged that males have lower requirements than this, but over one tenth of women – those with relatively high menstrual blood losses – have higher needs.

Food Sources

Liver, beef, offal, eggs
Wholemeal bread, wheat bran, fortified breakfast cereals
Dried apricots, figs, raisins and prunes
Soya beans
Spinach, broccoli, potatoes
Blackstrap molasses can provide 1.5mg iron per 7g teaspoon

Food Factors Influencing Iron Uptake

There are two forms of iron in the diet. Haem iron – an organically bound form found in animal sources, is relatively easily absorbed. Non-haem iron – an inorganic form found in vegetable sources, is less readily absorbed. The absorption of iron from vegetable sources is improved by vitamin C (e.g. from orange juice), which can increase its uptake by up to a third.

If you are a tea addict, then beware! Excessive amounts of tea provide tannic acid which reacts with non-haem iron, reducing its absorption. Phosphoric acid in fizzy pop may also have the same effect; as may phytic acid, from wheat bran.

Choosing An Iron Supplement

If you are pregnant or think you are anaemic, see your doctor, as you may need more iron than is available in supplements over the counter.

However, over-the-counter iron supplements can be used as an insurance by teenagers, vegetarians, menstruating women, after illness, or in the elderly. They can be purchased as a variety of compounds, but it is well known that some individuals can be sensitive to certain iron compounds, usually ferrous sulphate. This is a relatively poorly absorbed inorganic iron, and those that have a sensitivity to it complain of nausea or constipation. Ferrous sulphate is sometimes the form of iron used in multivitamin plus-iron products, so check the ingredients list on the label.

Organic iron compounds such as ferrous gluconate and ferrous fumarate are likely to be better tolerated, and amino acid chelated iron supplements are also well tolerated as they contain iron in a form similar to the well-absorbed haem iron.

You can also get organic iron in liquid tonic form, suitable as a general pick-me-up, and ideal for the elderly or youngsters, who can't swallow tablets or capsules. A daily dosage normally provides 7mg–10mg. Always follow the instructions very carefully though.

Buying Tips

For a better-tolerated iron supplement, make sure the iron is supplied as an organic compound. Always avoid 'ferric' compounds of iron, as these are the worst absorbed of all (check labels).

Look out for iron supplements that also contain vitamin C. This vitamin promotes the absorption of non-haem iron from the diet.

Safety

If you have not specifically been diagnosed as iron deficient, don't take more than 15mg iron daily, as an excess may promote certain oxidation processes in your body that could be potentially harmful. A doctor will advise how much iron you need if you are anaemic.

High intakes of certain types of iron may turn faeces a blackish colour.

Most cases of iron toxicity relate to accidental overload in young children. Iron supplements should always be kept well out of the way of children, and many manufacturers are now using childproof caps on supplements containing iron.

Iron Mini-File
- *Needed for healthy red blood cells*
- *A deficiency leads to anaemia (tiredness, etc.)*
- *More needed by menstruating women*
- *Extra may be required in pregnancy*
- *Most easily absorbed from meat sources*
- *Vitamin C improves absorption from vegetable sources*
- *Supplements containing organic compounds are better absorbed*
- *EC RDA = 14mg*

Magnesium

Magnesium is a vital component of bones and teeth, and is sometimes known as the 'anti-stress' mineral because of its close connection with the nervous system.

What Does It Do?

Over a half of the body's magnesium is found in our bones, where, along with calcium and phosphorus, it provides skeletal structure and strength.

Magnesium is a co-factor in energy-producing reactions, and so is closely involved in energy release. It is also important in the correct functioning of our nerves and muscles. A lack of this mineral may lead to increased irritability, anxiety, or even mild depression. Eyelid or facial twitches, 'restless leg syndrome' and other muscle spasms may sometimes indicate a lack of magnesium.

Magnesium is also closely involved with the body's use of calcium. Along with vitamin B6, magnesium helps to ensure calcium is correctly deposited in bones, and not in blood vessels or the kidneys.

Magnesium supplements are sometimes useful in women who suffer premenstrual cramps or sugar cravings. Magnesium has a role in regulating blood sugar levels, and tests show blood levels of the mineral may fall before menstruation.

As magnesium is involved in the pumping of the heart muscle, low levels can sometimes result in palpitations. Some heart attack victims are treated with magnesium sulphate injections in hospital.

A small study, reported in the *Lancet* (1991), indicated that magnesium seemed to reduce muscle pain and increase energy levels in ME sufferers, but this has yet to be corroborated with other evidence.

How Much Do We Need?

The EC Recommended Daily Allowance (RDA) for magnesium is 300mg; the average intake by women in the UK is 237mg per day. The body finds magnesium one of the hardest minerals to absorb from the diet.

Food Sources

Nuts (especially brazils)

Wholemeal bread, brown rice

Raisins, dried figs, dried apricots

Potatoes, peas

Two slices of wholemeal bread supply around 70mg of magnesium.

Note: Milk is a rich source of calcium, but a poor source of magnesium.

Choosing A Magnesium Supplement

Magnesium is available at dosages of 50mg–200mg per tablet or capsule, with recommended intakes usually being up to 300mg or so per day. Magnesium carbonate (found in dolomite tablets), and magnesium oxide, are common sources of this mineral, but they are inorganic, and don't tend to be as well absorbed as organic sources, e.g. gluconates, citrates and amino acid chelates (*see* Absorbing Minerals, p. 69).

Magnesium formulations may contain the useful co-nutrient vitamin B6; those aimed at bone health are usually combinations of magnesium with calcium and perhaps vitamin D. Magnesium may also be a central constituent of some 'premenstrual' supplements.

Safety

There is no evidence that large intakes of magnesium are harmful in healthy people. Up to 350mg daily as a supplement is thought to be safe.

Magnesium Mini-File ─────────────────────

- *Helps maintain strong bones*
- *Closely linked with calcium*

- *May help reduce muscle twitches*
- *With B6, may reduce risk of kidney stones*
- *May be helpful in PMS*
- *Needed for heart health*
- *EC RDA = 300mg*

Boron

Boron is a trace mineral only found to be important for humans since the 1980s. Our bones contain the highest amounts of this mineral. There are only a few studies examining boron's effects, but initial research suggests that boron can slow down calcium and magnesium loss from the bones in menopausal/post-menopausal women. Other evidence suggests boron may benefit some forms of arthritis.

Vegetables, nuts, soya, and dried fruit are the best dietary sources of boron. As a food supplement, up to 3mg of boron is safe to take on a daily basis. A number of supplements formulated for menopausal women, or for bone strength, include some boron.

Zinc

Zinc compounds are often found in nappy rash creams and rust-proofing paints, but zinc is also a vital mineral for our health and well being. The nutrient has been identified as being essential to over eighty bodily processes.

What Does it Do?

Zinc is an antioxidant mineral needed for a healthy immune defence system, and for repair and renewal of skin cells. A diet marginally lacking in zinc can lead to problems such as frequent infections, delayed wound healing, reduced appetite, decreased sense of taste and smell, poor skin condition and white flecks on the nails.

A very severe zinc deficiency leads to stunting and poor sexual development – first noted in Egyptian males in the 1950s. Such drastically low levels of zinc are not seen in this country, but some groups – particularly young women between 16 and 24 – do often have lower than desirable intakes.

Professor Bryce-Smith, Professor of Organic Chemistry at Reading University, has done pioneering work into the relationship between zinc and the slimmer's disease anorexia nervosa. His observations have led him to suspect that zinc deficiency contributes to the anorexic condition by impairing the sense of taste and smell, and therefore the desire to eat. He has used zinc as part of treatment programmes for anorexia nervosa victims.

Zinc is also important for reproductive health. Low zinc levels may result in reduced sperm count, and pregnant women with low blood levels of zinc may give birth to smaller babies. Poor growth in the first few months of life has been associated with declining levels of zinc in breast milk.

Men have a high concentration of zinc in their prostate gland, and many anecdotal reports indicate that benign enlargement of the prostate gland – causing increased frequency of urination in middle aged men – can be improved by consuming extra zinc.

Zinc is also commonly taken as a supplement to help with skin conditions such as acne or eczema. The basis of zinc therapy lies in the fact that the mineral is necessary for normal cell division, tissue repair and renewal. Zinc is also necessary for the metabolism of fatty acids into important substances which help regulate our skin health.

Some clinical studies have also found that zinc (sucked as lozenges) helps cold symptoms, whilst others have shown no conclusive result.

How Much Do We Need?

The EC Recommended Daily Allowance (RDA) for zinc is 15mg. The Dietary and Nutritional Survey of British Adults (HMSO, 1990) found the average daily intake was lower than this at 11.4mg for men and 8.4mg for women.

Food Sources

Oysters
Liver, meat
Shrimps, sardines
Nuts, seeds, wholemeal bread
Eggs, cheese

Choosing A Supplement

Zinc can be taken as part of a multivitamin and mineral formulation, or separately. Multinutrient formulations contain a wide variety of levels – anything from 1mg–15mg. 5mg–10mg zinc daily is ideal for topping up the dietary level of this mineral, whereas 15mg is more likely to be taken for guarding against colds or to help in skin conditions.

Inorganic forms of zinc such as zinc sulphate, carbonate or zinc oxide may not be as well absorbed as organic forms such as gluconate, citrate or zinc chelated with amino acids. Zinc picolinate is closely related to amino acid chelated zinc, and may be particularly well absorbed. Check labels to see how the zinc appears. Also look for zinc in antioxidant formulations. You would expect to see 10mg–15mg in these types of product.

Zinc lozenges are sometimes available, and are of most use if you actually feel a cold or sore throat coming on. They have a local action, and are usually found in dosages of 3.5mg–7mg per lozenge.

Buying Tips

If you are purchasing a separate zinc supplement for long term daily use, choose one that also contains a little copper. Copper is an essential mineral that can be depleted by prolonged zinc intake.

Safety

Zinc is not in itself unsafe, but high intakes (above 30mg) may deplete or unbalance other nutrients in the body – namely copper, iron and possibly folic acid. Erring on the side of caution, the Ministry of Agriculture, Fisheries and Food has asked responsible supplements manufacturers not to supply products containing more than 15mg zinc in a daily dose. More than 15mg of supplemental zinc daily should not be taken, except on the advice of a qualified practitioner.

Zinc Mini-File

- *Needed for a healthy skin*
- *Important for reproductive health*
- *High concentration in prostate gland*
- *Lozenges may be sucked at first sign of a cold*
- *Needed for sense of taste and smell*
- *EC RDA = 15mg*

Selenium

Selenium has been known as an essential trace mineral – needed to prevent degeneration of liver tissue – for only two decades. About half of the body's 5mg–10mg of selenium is found in the liver.

Dietary sources of selenium vary widely across the world,

according to the soil content of this mineral. In Finland, where soil selenium is naturally very low, selenium is added to fertilisers and to animal feed. Most of Britain has low levels of soil selenium.

What Does It Do?

Selenium forms part of a key antioxidant enzyme, glutathione peroxidase, which helps to protect the fatty parts of our cells from going rancid (*see* Antioxidants, p. 64).

Many selenium functions are closely linked with vitamin E; the two have a synergistic (complementary) relationship. For example, selenium, with vitamin E, is involved in our antibody response to harmful germs, and so can help maintain our immune system.

There is now good evidence, from the USA, Finland and China, that low selenium levels in the body are linked to an increased risk of cancer and heart disease. Cancer sufferers tend to have selenium levels around 30% lower than the norm for healthy people.

Selenium also helps the body produce anti-inflammatory prostaglandins (hormone-like substances), and so some rheumatoid arthritis sufferers find taking extra selenium helpful.

The mineral is required for the production of thyroxine, a hormone made by the thyroid gland which helps regulate metabolic rate.

How Much Do We Need?

At present, there is no EC Recommended Daily Allowance for selenium, but the Department of Health Reference Nutrient Intake (RNI) is 60 microgrammes per day for adult females and 75 microgrammes a day for adult males.

Vegetarians, the elderly, those on a 'junk food' diet, smokers and pregnant/nursing mothers are groups at risk from low selenium levels.

Research has shown that up to 200 microgrammes a day may

be needed to effectively reduce fat rancidity – which is linked with heart disease – in the blood.

Food Sources

Liver, kidney, and other meat
Fish, shellfish (shrimps, crab)
Wholemeal bread, wholegrains (depending on country of origin)
Dairy products

Choosing A Selenium Supplement

Most selenium supplements come in strengths of 100 or 200 microgrammes (μg). Vitamin E reinforces the action of selenium and is normally included as well, and some products also include zinc or vitamin C as supporting antioxidants. Some multivitamin formulations may include small amounts of selenium which are intended to make good any deficiency in the diet rather than to have any therapeutic effect.

In food, selenium is only found in its organic form, and this is the best form for supplements. Look for selenium yeast (as long as you don't have a yeast allergy), amino acid chelated selenium, or, best of all, seleno-methionine. These are well absorbed; sodium selenite and sodium selenate are inorganic forms of selenium that are not as well absorbed.

Selenium And Arthritis

There is a popular belief that selenium can ease the pain and misery of arthritis, and there is some anecdotal evidence to back this view. When a health magazine offered supplements containing 100 microgrammes of selenium to 1000 participants in a free trial, improvement of arthritis was one of the main claimed benefits. No distinction was made between types of the disease, but it is thought that rheumatoid arthritis is more likely to be responsive to selenium than osteoarthritis.

Selenium levels have generally been found to be depressed in arthritis sufferers, and although more studies are needed, one 1992 *British Journal of Rheumatology* report found that a daily 200 microgramme selenium supplement did give definite improvements in the progress of some sufferers.

Safety

Taking supplements of up to 200 microgrammes on a daily basis is considered quite safe for adults. Intakes of five times this amount, i.e. 1mg, for a period of two years have been known to cause nausea and nail and hair changes.

Selenium Mini-File

- *Widely used as an antioxidant*
- *Vitamin E reinforces action of selenium*
- *May help reduce risk of heart disease and cancer*
- *Arthritis sufferers may benefit from selenium*
- *Helps strengthen immune system*
- *Preserves normal liver function*

Chromium

Chromium may be better known for its use in plating metals, but it is also an essential mineral in the diet. Chromium exists in two chemical forms – the 'trivalent' form is active as a nutrient, whereas the 'hexavalent' form is treated differently by the body, and can be toxic.

What Does It Do?

Chromium is an important part of an organic complex called glucose tolerance factor (GTF). GTF is made up of chromium in association with niacin (vitamin B3) and various amino acids, and its function is to increase the effectiveness of insulin, a hormone which helps regulate blood sugar levels.

Severe chromium deficiency is known to result in poor glucose tolerance, the precursor to diabetic conditions. A highly refined diet, with a large intake of sugars that require chromium for metabolism, could predispose some individuals to a chromium deficiency and aggravate adult-onset diabetes. Because of its role in the regulation of blood glucose levels, chromium is often taken as a supplement by people who crave sugary foods, e.g. sweets and chocolate.

Chromium has been advocated as a sports supplement, on the basis that it potentiates insulin which encourages the uptake of amino acids (protein) into muscle. However its effectiveness in this area has yet to be reliably proven.

Chromium might also play a role in maintaining a healthy low cholesterol level in the blood. When glucose tolerance is impaired – a possible consequence of chromium deficiency – the liver manufactures more cholesterol; so maintaining an adequate intake of chromium could be important for a healthy heart.

How Much Do We Need?

Chromium does not have a Recommended Daily Allowance (RDA), but it's thought that an intake above 20 microgrammes daily is not likely to be associated with any deficiency symptoms. American authorities suggest a 'safe and adequate' intake of between 50 and 200 microgrammes daily.

Food Sources

Whole grains, Brewer's yeast
Hard water
Meat, kidneys
Cheese

Choosing A Supplement

A few microgrammes of chromium may be present in multi-vitamin and mineral formulations, but chromium supplements also exist in their own right, usually at strengths of 100 or 200 microgrammes. The mineral may be presented as chromium picolinate or amino acid chelated chromium, both of which provide the safer trivalent form of chromium. However, chromium yeast is thought to provide the mineral predominantly as GTF – which is particularly well absorbed by the body. Chromium polynicotinate, a yeast-free version of chromium, also closely mimics how the mineral occurs in the GTF complex.

Safety

No adverse effects have been noted from the intake of supplements containing trivalent chromium, although certain doubts as to the long term safety of high levels of chromium picolinate have yet to be resolved. A safe level for self-supplementation with chromium is up to 200 microgrammes per day.

Caution: If you are an insulin-dependent diabetic, it is recommended that you do not take individual chromium supplements without a doctor's advice.

Chromium Mini-File

- *Part of glucose tolerance factor*
- *Helps in regulation of blood sugar levels*
- *May help maintain healthy cholesterol levels*
- *Sometimes taken by sports people*

CHAPTER FOUR

Other Common Food Supplements

Fish Oil

Since spoonfuls of cod liver oil were given to wartime babies, the consumption of fish oil has remained a strong tradition in Britain. Whilst the market for fish oil supplements is very strong, there is much confusion surrounding the number of different product types available.

What Does It Do?

Fish oil is a term encompassing both liver oils (obtained from the liver of white fish such as cod and halibut) and fish oil concentrate (obtained from the flesh of oily fish such as salmon). Cod liver oil supplements are rich in vitamins A and D, and contain variable amounts of the important fatty acids eicosapentaenoic acid (EPA) and docosahexaenoic acid (DHA); however supplements of fish oil concentrate are rich in EPA and DHA but do not contain vitamins A or D.

EPA is an active ingredient of fish oil involved in producing important hormone-like substances called prostaglandins. The prostaglandins produced from EPA help to:

1 Reduce the stickiness of the blood, making it less liable to clot and cause thrombosis.

2   Reduce levels of 'triglyceride' blood fats.

3   Modestly reduce blood pressure when it is raised.

These combined effects, together with a low fat diet and healthy lifestyle, could result in a reduced risk of cardiovascular disease. In one study (*Lancet*, 1989), 2–3 fish meals a week, or an intake of EPA and DHA from a supplement, significantly reduced mortality in men who had already had one heart attack.

The prostaglandins made from EPA also have the property of being less inflammatory than those made from other fatty acids in the diet. It is thought that EPA-rich fish oils may therefore have a mild anti-inflammatory effect – possibly helping to relieve conditions such as psoriasis, inflammatory bowel problems and arthritis.

In fact arthritis sufferers are the most common consumers of EPA-rich fish oils. A number of studies have shown that the need for non-steroidal anti-inflammatory drugs (such as ibuprofen) is reduced in rheumatoid arthritis patients taking several capsules of fish oil concentrate daily. Fish oil may be able to reduce the symptoms of rheumatoid arthritis – tender joints, morning stiffness and swelling – but it is not a cure.

Osteoarthritis, which is simple wear and tear on joints experienced with ageing, is less likely to respond to fish oils. However, if there is inflammation, some benefit may still be experienced.

How Much Do We Need?

Currently, our combined intake of EPA and DHA is only around 1g per week, but the British Nutrition Foundation, in its 1993 briefing paper 'Nutritional Aspects of Fish', recommended that we should be consuming eight to ten times this – an amount roughly equivalent to at least:

- 1–2 servings of fatty fish a week (mackerel, herring, salmon, pilchards, sardines)

- or: 1 teaspoon cod liver oil daily
- or: 4 x 1g fish oil concentrate capsules daily

Any combination of the above could of course be consumed to achieve the desirable intake of EPA and DHA.

Choosing A Fish Oil Supplement

Before buying a fish oil supplement, you must decide what you want to take it for. If you require the Recommended Daily Allowance (RDA) of vitamins A and D to help maintain healthy bones, skin, mucous passages (e.g. respiratory tract) and immune system, the most basic cod liver oil or halibut liver oil capsules will provide this.

However, if you want fish oil to help maintain a healthy heart, or to help with rheumatic joints, make sure to read the label and ensure that EPA and DHA are listed. If you don't eat much fish, particularly fatty fish, the minimum combined quantity of EPA and DHA that is likely to be effective is around 1000mg per day.

Content Of Major Fish Oil Product Types

Product	EPA/DHA Level	Vitamins A and D?
Halibut liver oil caps	Negligible	Yes
1-a-day cod liver oil caps (regular)	Negligible	Yes
1-a-day cod liver oil caps (high strength)	Low	Yes
Cod liver oil (liquid)	High	Yes
Fish oil concentrate caps	Medium*	No

*Fish oil concentrate provides around 300mg combined EPA and DHA per 1000mg capsule. A few products may have been chemically altered to provide even higher amounts.

Buying Tips

Check labels carefully for vitamin A and D content (needed for healthy bones, teeth and mucous passages), and/or EPA and DHA content (helps joints and heart). Remember that most inexpensive 'one-a-day' cod liver oil capsules only provide vitamins A and D in useful amounts. They are not rich in EPA and DHA – and so can't be used to help arthritic joints!

Fish Oils And Early Brain Development

DHA – a fatty acid found only in fish oils – is a vital component of brain tissue, and increases steadily in the foetal brain during the last three months of pregnancy. Failure to accumulate DHA at this time has been shown to impair the child's learning ability, so pregnant and lactating women should try to ensure a good dietary intake of oily fish (or take fish oil concentrate capsules). For vegetarians, DHA can be made in the body from linolenic acid – found in linseed and rapeseed oils.

Safety

Cod liver oil contains vitamins A and D which in large excess can be toxic. So don't take more cod liver oil than recommended, and watch when you are combining it with other supplements that may provide vitamins A and D, particularly if you are pregnant. (*See* Vitamin and Mineral Safety, p. 20, 21.) Very large amounts of EPA and DHA may thin the blood, so if you are taking anti-coagulant medication (e.g. warfarin or daily low dose aspirin), speak to your doctor before taking anything other than regular amounts of fish oil.

_____ ***Fish Oil Mini-File***

Fish oil concentrate capsules/liquid cod liver oil:
- *Provide fatty acids EPA and DHA*
- *May help maintain a healthy heart*
- *May be useful in arthritic conditions*
- *Cod liver oil also provides vitamin A and D*
- *Maintain healthy bones, skin and mucous passages and build resistance to minor infections*

Cod liver oil/halibut liver oil capsules:
- *Provide vitamins A and D*
- *Usually provide negligible or small amounts of EPA and DHA*

Evening Primrose Oil

Evening primrose oil is the oil obtained from the seeds of the evening primrose plant (no relation to our native wild primrose). The oil contains a very unusual fatty acid (component of fat) called gamma linolenic acid (GLA). There are no normal dietary sources of this fatty acid, and we normally have to make it from another fatty acid called linoleic acid, which is widely obtainable in vegetable oils.

What Does It Do?

Evening primrose oil provides a direct source of GLA which can prove beneficial in people who have difficulty in making this fatty acid from linoleic acid. Factors which have been suggested as blocking the body's natural production of GLA include viruses (e.g. colds, flu), stress, alcohol, saturated fats, ageing and a lack of certain nutrients.

GLA is needed for the manufacture of certain hormone-like regulatory substances called prostaglandins. Research has shown that the prostaglandins made from GLA can have beneficial regulatory effects on the immune system, circulation and the menstrual cycle.

Many women take evening primrose oil prior to menstruation (*see* page 98). It is also popular as a supplement during the menopause, although a study in the *British Medical Journal* (1994) found no significant benefit in hot flushes. However, many women do find evening primrose oil helpful at the change of life, possibly because its active ingredient (GLA) may help in promoting hormone balance.

Evening primrose oil also helps in maintaining good skin condition, partly by providing fatty acids which help maintain skin cell membranes which 'lock in' moisture. Many women take evening primrose oil simply because they find it improves the smoothness of skin, enhances hair lustre and strengthens nails.

Evening primrose oil has also been documented to help the irritation in the more serious skin affliction, eczema. Some doctors prescribe it for this condition, but the level used can be high. However, lower levels may help, depending on the severity and underlying cause. Other nutrients, such as zinc and vitamin A, may also play a role in managing eczema.

It's thought that evening primrose oil may help to dampen down the overreaction of the immune system that can be at the root of atopic (allergic) conditions such as eczema. That's why evening primrose may also be recommended in rheumatoid arthritis, where it's thought the body's own immune system begins attacking the joints.

A study at Glasgow Royal Infirmary (1988), found that evening primrose oil helped sufferers reduce their anti-rheumatic drugs, especially in conjunction with fish oils. The Arthritis and Rheumatism Council acknowledge that evening primrose oil and fish oil may be helpful when incorporated as part of a healthy diet.

Evening primrose oil is sometimes also recommended in

multiple sclerosis to correct a fatty acid imbalance often seen in the disease; this usage should be discussed with your doctor.

How Much Should I Take?

Many people don't get results with evening primrose oil because they don't take enough to give the benefit that's expected. 500mg–1000mg daily may be fine as a purely cosmetic supplement, but you'll need more if you have severe PMS, rheumatoid arthritis or eczema. In fact the minimum amount that seems to have any effect in these situations is around 2000mg. You'll also need to persevere for at least three or four months before you can make a proper decision as to whether it is effective.

Choosing An Evening Primrose Oil Supplement

In evening primrose oil, 8%–10% of the total oil is made up of GLA, so you'd expect a 500mg product claiming '10% GLA' to have 50mg of this fatty acid per capsule. However, some products actually provide a few milligrammes less than this, because the GLA content is given as 'percentage of total fatty acids' – which make up less than 100% of the oil. Check labels!

If you are concerned about environmental issues, you may wish to find out how the oil has been extracted. Some evening primrose products are made by extracting the oil from the seeds with solvents, whilst others are made by mechanically pressing the oil from the seed.

Some evening primrose oil products make a 'cold pressed' claim. Whilst cold pressing may be desirable for cooking oil where retention of flavour and aroma is important, it is of no relevance or nutritional advantage in evening primrose taken as a supplement.

Evening primrose oil may also be included at low levels in certain cod liver oil or multivitamin products. If you want benefits from evening primrose oil, you are best to take it as an individual supplement.

However, evening primrose oil may sometimes be mixed in beneficial quantities with fish oil concentrate in multi-dose capsules. These are aimed primarily at maintaining heart health and joint mobility.

Evening primrose oil may occasionally be provided as chewable tablets or liquid, but these are more expensive than capsules.

Buying Tips

Choose a formulation that also provides vitamin E. This vitamin protects polyunsaturated fats – of the type provided by evening primrose oil – from oxidation in the body. It makes nutritional sense to take the two together, but note no evening primrose oil product contains high levels of vitamin E by supplement standards (typically 5mg–10mg per 500mg capsule).

Link evening primrose oil with a multivitamin if your diet isn't what it could be. The efficacy of evening primrose oil depends on certain co-factor nutrients needed to further process GLA in the body.

Evening Primrose Oil And PMS

There are some anecdotal reports, and a few trials, attesting to the benefits of evening primrose oil in premenstrual syndrome. In one pilot study, evening primrose oil was taken daily by women in the two weeks leading up to their period, with very good results. Of these women, 95% noted improvements in abdomen and breast discomfort, 80% reported that they were less irritable, 79% found the swelling in their fingers and ankles reduced, and more than half were less anxious.

In another study, 61% of PMS patients reported complete relief, and 35% partial relief, with evening primrose oil.

Whilst a benefit has yet to be proved in larger scale studies of generalised PMS symptoms, evening primrose oil does excel itself in the specific relief of premenstrual breast pain, and also in benign breast cysts.

For potential results in PMS, at least 1500mg–2000mg evening primrose oil should be taken daily in the two weeks leading up to menstruation. Sometimes, up to 4g (4000mg) may be required.

Starflower Oil

Starflower (borage) oil is an even richer source of GLA than evening primrose oil, containing around 22% GLA (of total oil). Consequently, less needs to be consumed to provide a given quantity of GLA. Starflower oil is available singly, or may be combined in evening primrose oil products.

However the chemical structure of starflower oil is quite different from that of evening primrose oil, and some scientists have therefore questioned whether it is as effective a source of GLA as evening primrose oil. Certainly it is true to say that the health benefits of evening primrose oil have been more widely researched: more studies on starflower oil will help to clarify its comparative efficacy.

Also, contrary to popular opinion, starflower oil work out as a more expensive way of obtaining GLA than evening primrose oil. Do the calculations!

Safety

Evening primrose oil is very safe, but excessive levels may help thin the blood, so never take more than the recommended dosage if you take warfarin or a similar anticoagulant drug. Evening primrose oil may also be best avoided by some epileptics or schizophrenics – check with your doctor before taking.

Evening Primrose Oil Mini-File

- *Provides gamma linolenic acid (GLA)*
- *Can improve skin condition*
- *Sometimes beneficial in PMS*
- *May help in rheumatoid arthritis*
- *Useful daily dosage around 2000mg*

Lecithin

Lecithin comprises a group of fatty substances which are made internally by the liver and are present in certain foods. Although found in all cells, large amounts of lecithin are found in the human brain – 40% of the brain is composed of lecithin in the form of phosphatidyl ('phos-fa-tidal') choline. Lecithin is widely used as an emulsifier in food products, e.g. margarine and chocolate bars, helping to combine oil- and water-based ingredients.

What Does It Do?

The components of lecithin include phosphatidyl choline, phosphorus, choline, inositol and polyunsaturated fatty acids such as linoleic acid. Lecithin helps maintain the structure of cell membranes, and is involved in the transport of fats in the body.

The capacity of bile (involved in fat digestion) to emulsify cholesterol depends on lecithin, and high levels may therefore help reduce the risk of gallstones in susceptible people. Gallstone sufferers often have a low ratio of lecithin to cholesterol, and extra lecithin helps to normalise this balance.

There is no strong evidence that lecithin can lower blood cholesterol levels, but if it is to have an effect, very high doses are likely to be needed, together with a low-fat, antioxidant-rich diet.

Lecithin is a good source of choline, a close 'cousin' of the water soluble B vitamins. Choline is needed to make acetylcholine, a neurotransmitter (brain chemical) essential for normal brain activity. Some naturopathic practitioners recommend high levels of lecithin to help slow down deleterious brain changes in those suffering from dementia-type illnesses.

Choline, along with another lecithin component, inositol, also helps prevent fat accumulation in the wrong places. For example, choline has been shown to help clear excess fat deposits from the liver.

Additionally, choline helps to maintain the myelin sheath, which insulates the nerves. There is some evidence that this becomes depleted in MS (multiple sclerosis) sufferers, and that lecithin or choline supplements may help slow down this deterioration.

Food Sources

Soya beans, egg yolk
Liver, meat, trout
Wholegrains, peanuts, wheatgerm, beans and peas

Choosing A Lecithin Supplement

2g–3g is the amount of lecithin often recommended as a daily supplement. For example this amount is sometimes advocated as helpful in preventing the formation of gallstones, although this has yet to be proven.

Most lecithin supplements are produced from soya beans, and lecithin capsules are generally found in 200mg, 600mg or 1200mg strengths. You would need to take a lot of the 200mg-size per day to produce a worthwhile effect, so most people opt for the latter strengths.

Lecithin granules, which can be sprinkled on food, are also available and are a rich source. The granules can be used to obtain much higher intakes of lecithin, e.g. for more specific health problems, or as directed by a practitioner.

Separate choline and inositol supplements are sometimes also available.

Safety
There are no reported side effects from lecithin, even at very high intakes.

> *Lecithin Mini-File* _____
> - *Important fat emulsifier*
> - *Required for proper cell membrane structure*
> - *May help brain health in the elderly*
> - *Reduces certain fatty deposits in the liver*
> - *Rich source of choline and inositol, related to B complex vitamins*
> - *2g–3g daily is the normal supplemental intake*

Garlic

Garlic is a herb that has been used throughout the ages. It is said that it was consumed by the Egyptian pyramid builders and, in the First World War, crushed garlic was applied to soldiers' wounds for its antiseptic qualities. Nowadays, some of garlic's traditional uses are being proved by research.

What Does It Do?
Garlic has an established track record as a protection against colds and minor infections, and particularly for helping to relieve

catarrh. More recently, garlic's effects on the heart have been studied – it is now established that incorporated in a healthy low fat diet, garlic can have a beneficial effect on cholesterol levels, blood pressure and the stickiness of blood.

Garlic supplements are often taken by people suffering from an overgrowth of the yeast organism Candida albicans. Recent research has also indicated that some garlic preparations may act as a cell-protective antioxidant.

The key beneficial compounds in garlic are thought to be a variety of water and oil soluble sulphur compounds. Oil soluble compounds are smelly, whilst water soluble compounds tend not to have an odour.

Garlic has also been found to have unique non-sulphur compounds, which also make an important contribution to garlic's health benefits.

Unlike most other foods, processing can actually improve the benefits of garlic. It triggers the formation of a cascade of compounds that do not already exist in raw garlic – different forms of processing result in different compounds being formed.

Understanding Garlic

A quick look at the basic chemistry of garlic can help to appreciate the differences between garlic supplements.

An intact garlic clove contains a sulphur compound called alliin, which is odourless. It is only when you cut or crush a garlic clove that alliin comes into contact with an enzyme called alliinase, and the substance called allicin is then formed. Allicin acts as a natural insecticide for the garlic bulb. It is very unstable and quickly starts being converted into a variety of other compounds, which contribute to the beneficial effects of garlic.

Types Of Garlic Supplement

Garlic Oils

Garlic oil capsules provide essential oil of garlic diluted in a base of vegetable oil. The essential oil is usually steamed distilled from the garlic, the cloves yielding a small amount of concentrated oil. Hence garlic oil products tend to be only a few milligrammes in strength, typically 0.66mg, 2mg or 4mg per capsule. Garlic oil products may provide some symptomatic relief in cases of colds and catarrh.

About 4mg garlic oil daily can bring about some beneficial effects on the cardiovascular system, but up to 12mg gives better results (according to research presented at the 67th session of the American Heart Association, 1994).

Unfortunately, garlic oil, which mainly contains oily sulphides, is also a potent source of garlic odour. However, odour masking can be achieved by modifying the capsule shell, or by adding peppermint or parsley. Garlic oil may also be slightly irritant if you have a sensitive digestive system.

Macerates

Macerated garlic products are made by steeping mashed raw garlic in vegetable oil, and encapsulating the resultant mixture. They can be rich in particular oil soluble sulphur components, but tend to be very smelly in use. A simpler version is made by mixing just a few milligrammes of ordinary garlic powder with vegetable oil – making a very weak garlic supplement.

Powdered Tablets or Capsules

These products are made from whole garlic which has been dried and powdered. (Two thirds of a fresh garlic clove is made up of water.)

Some powdered garlic products are designed to release allicin in the intestines. The cloves have to be sliced carefully and dried before making into tablets, so that some alliinase enzyme is left unreacted (*see* above). Allicin should then be made in the body upon consumption of the supplement – followed by further metabolism into active garlic substances. However, it's vital that the product has a special 'enteric coat' to let it reach the intestines before breaking down. This is because alliinase, the enzyme needed to make allicin can be destroyed by stomach acid.

A suitable daily dosage of powdered garlic is around 600mg a day, or as directed. At this sort of level, products that release allicin in the intestines have been shown to help in maintaining healthy cholesterol levels and blood pressure.

Aged Garlic Extract

Aged garlic extract contains large amounts of odourless water soluble compounds and relatively smaller amounts of oil-soluble compounds. As such it has the advantage of being a very sociable garlic product!

Aged garlic extract is made by crushing fresh garlic and allowing it to 'age' in large tanks for around 20 months. During the ageing process, alliin and allicin are gradually 'bioconverted' into a range of sulphur-containing compounds which are non-irritant and odourless. This means that these important garlic-derived substances are already preformed in the product.

Studies are currently taking place regarding the antifungal effect of aged garlic extract when applied topically in athlete's foot. It is also widely used in America to help guard against the effects of pollution and to help maintain a healthy heart and cholesterol balance.

Aged garlic is available in tablet dosages from 100mg–600mg. 100mg–300mg is a lower daily 'maintenance' level; 1000mg may be needed for more specific health benefits.

Choosing A Supplement

All types of garlic supplement can bring benefits, but they are prepared in many different ways, so don't expect to compare strengths across product types. Use the individual descriptions listed above to get an indication of which dosage may be beneficial and the pros and cons of each product type.

Buying Tips

Remember – you cannot compare garlic oil capsules with tablet formulations when looking at strengths.

Garlic Mini-File

- *May help fight colds and flu*
- *Useful in catarrh*
- *May help maintain a healthy heart*
- *May benefit people with Candida albicans infection*
- *Higher levels help reduce cholesterol levels*

Lactic Bacteria

Lactic bacteria are 'friendly' micro-organisms which transform sugars into lactic acid via a process called fermentation. They are very abundant in nature and are used in the food industry for the production of yoghurts and other fermented milk products.

What Do They Do?

Lactic bacteria protect the gut against certain disease-causing bacteria, assist in the final digestion of food, and help maintain the natural acidity of the vagina.

Lactic gut bacteria assist in defending us against infection by maintaining an acidic microclimate that harmful bacteria cannot thrive in, and forming a physical barrier which stops them from 'sticking' to the gut wall and multiplying. Studies have also shown that supplements of lactic bacteria may inhibit the action of certain enzymes that promote the formation of toxins in the bowel.

A healthy balance of lactic bacteria in the gut will also help inhibit the overgrowth of fungal organisms such as Candida albicans (*see* page 110), and together with a healthy, high fibre diet, may help promote normal bowel action.

Supplements of lactic bacteria may also help reduce a minor intolerance to lactose (milk sugar) – characterised by gastric symptoms on consuming dairy products – through converting the lactose to lactic acid.

Although our individual gut flora normally remains quite constant, certain factors may deplete or modify the harmony of intestinal bacteria. Such factors include use of broad spectrum antibiotics, the contraceptive pill or steroids; chronic constipation, diarrhoea or consumption of contaminated foods.

Lactobacilli And Bifidobacteria

There are different families of lactic bacteria, the two main ones being Lactobacilli and Bifidobacteria. Examples of lactobacilli include L. acidophilus, L. rhamnosus and L. casei, and examples of Bifidobacteria include B. bifidum and B. longum. Both families of 'friendly' bacteria can be found throughout the gut, but broadly speaking, Bifidobacteria – which cannot live in oxygen – are more predominant in the bowel than they are in the small intestine.

Lactobacillus bifidum – a name sometimes still used on supplement labels – is old terminology, indicating the presence of Bifidobacteria.

Storing and Using Lactic Bacteria

Lactic bacteria supplements provide 'friendly' bacteria in a state of 'suspended animation'. Warm, humid atmospheres need to be avoided during storage, as these will lead to a reduction in the number of viable bacteria. Most lactic bacteria supplements should therefore be kept in the refrigerator – especially those containing Bifidobacteria, which are particularly sensitive. Follow the manufacturer's instructions carefully.

The lactic bacteria in supplements are sensitive to stomach acid, so to reduce any potential losses before the supplement reaches the intestines, it is best to take the supplement straight after a meal, when the presence of food dilutes stomach acid. Milk or yogurt also act as particularly good protective mediums with which to consume lactic bacteria supplements.

What Is The Correct Dosage?

It is generally recognised that the minimum amount of lactic bacteria needed to have a good effect on gut health is one billion a day. However, more may be taken quite safely, and may be recommended in specific health conditions. (*Note:* One billion = one thousand million = 1,000,000,000.)

Choosing A Supplement

Lactic bacteria are most often taken to repopulate the gut after a course of antibiotics. A supplement may also be helpful after a stomach upset, or when exposed to different food and water (e.g. whilst travelling abroad). Many women on the contraceptive pill, or with a tendency to thrush, also take lactic bacteria supplements.

Most lactic bacteria supplements (tablets or capsules) claim to provide between half a billion and four billion bacteria in a daily dosage. Some products in powder form may provide more, but these tend to be the more specialist products for use under a practitioner's advice. Powder products also need to be more carefully used and stored, as contamination (e.g. through constantly dipping in a spoon) is easily possible.

Lactobacillus acidophilus is commonly used in supplements, but don't assume that because a product has a name ending '. . . dophilus' that it necessarily contains this strain. There are several strains of Lactobacilli that can be used in supplements, all of which are beneficial to digestive health.

Lactic bacteria products that contain Bifidobacteria may be more useful in terms of bowel health, whereas those purely based on Lactobacilli can be especially useful for intestinal or vaginal health.

Lactic bacteria supplements may also often contain maltodextrin, pectin, lactose, etc. as a food source for the bacteria, but the latter may be unsuitable for people with a dairy intolerance. The idea behind adding a food source is that the bacteria get immediate sustenance when they reach the gut, enabling them to reproduce more effectively. With the right conditions lactic bacteria can quickly multiply into billions and billions!

Adult lactic bacteria formulations may be used safely in youngsters, though a few specialist children's products may occasionally be available.

Buying Tips

If a lactic bacteria supplement says 'one billion bacteria at manufacture', you must bear in mind there will undoubtedly be less than this in the product, as there is an inevitable reduction in bacterial numbers during storage.

Lactic Bacteria And Thrush

Candida albicans is a fungal organism that lives in all of us. Most of the time it causes no symptoms, because it is kept at bay by the balance of other bacteria in the gut (or vagina). However, sometimes this balance may be upset, with the result that the Candida albicans organism grows out of control, causing symptoms such as bloating, digestive upset, poor skin condition, general malaise and vaginal or oral thrush.

A supplement of lactic bacteria, together with dietary modification (a low-sugar, and sometimes yeast-free diet) seem to be useful in helping to restore the balance of 'friendly' bacteria in the gut and vagina. Women on the contraceptive pill who frequently suffer from thrush often report that a supplement of lactic bacteria is useful to them; garlic may also be helpful.

Safety

Lactic bacteria are generally very safe when taken as a supplement.

Lactic Bacteria Mini-File
- *'Friendly' bacteria – Lactobacilli and Bifidobacteria*
- *Assist digestive processes*
- *Keep harmful bacteria at bay*
- *May help reduce symptoms of lactose intolerance*
- *Helpful to guard against Candida albicans ('thrush' organism)*
- *Minimum helpful intake = 1 billion per day*

Coenzyme Q10

Coenzyme Q10 is also known as a ubiquinone, from the Latin word meaning 'everywhere'. It is a naturally occurring fat-soluble substance found in every cell in the body, and was first discovered in 1957.

There are various coenzyme Q forms, but only coenzyme Q10 is important for the human body. Coenzyme Q10, or simply CoQ10, is made in the body, but production falls off as we age. CoQ10 is also found in foods, especially meat, but cooking and processing methods tend to destroy it.

What Does It Do?

Within each cell, CoQ10 helps create a substance called ATP (adenosine triphoshate). ATP is the energy source which 'sparks' or drives all the functions performed by the cell. Without CoQ10 there is no 'spark' to drive the cell's 'engine'. It is therefore not surprising to find the highest concentrations of CoQ10 in those organs which have the highest energy requirements, e.g. heart, muscles and liver.

A decline in these concentrations may mean the body's organs cannot meet their energy needs. It has been shown that heart patients tend to have low CoQ10 levels, and as the liver's ability to synthesise CoQ10 declines as we get older, a lack of energy in older people may, in part, be connected with lower CoQ10 production.

CoQ10 plays a part in our immune system, helping to stimulate certain white blood cells which are part of our 'immune army' fighting off invading germs; during and after illness we may need extra. CoQ10 also acts as an important antioxidant (cell protective) substance.

Heart patients and angina sufferers have in certain cases been shown to benefit from supplemental CoQ10 – it has been shown to improve cardiac output. This is thought to be due to an increase in oxygen utilisation by the heart muscle. Research in the USA and in Japan has shown that hypertension (high blood pressure) also responds well to CoQ10.

Another area of interest is oral health, where a lack of CoQ10 may be associated with periodontal (gum) disease. Some studies have shown that CoQ10 supplements can help diseased gums.

Food Sources
Sardines, mackerel and other fish
Meat, poultry, eggs
Wholegrains, nuts, peanut butter
Spinach, broccoli, vegetable oils

Choosing A CoQ10 Supplement
Supplements mainly come in 10mg, 15mg or 30mg strengths. A good starting level if you feel you may be low in CoQ10 is around 15mg daily. Signs may include unexplained tiredness (not related to lack of sleep or anaemia) and always feeling the cold. The elderly, vegetarians and vegans, and those who have been ill may be especially vulnerable to CoQ10 deficiency, and could benefit from its antioxidant- and immunity-enhancing properties.

Higher levels of CoQ10 (30mg plus) may be particularly useful in periodontal gum disease. You could also take it at this level to help support your heart function.

Buying Tips
Look out for CoQ10 in oil-based capsules – it may be better absorbed than from powdered formulations.

Safety
CoQ10 seems to be a safe nutrient, and has been used clinically at up to 150mg daily without any toxicity problems. However, early reports indicate that care may need to be taken with higher than normal doses if you are on blood thinning drugs such as warfarin.

CoQ10 Mini-File

- *Essential energy-releasing function*
- *Important antioxidant (cell protector)*
- *Made by the body*
- *Animal products are best food sources*
- *May be useful as we get older, or after illness*
- *May benefit heart conditions*
- *Helpful in gum disease*

Bee Products

Honey is the commonest product we obtain from bees, used as a food and natural sweetener. It is also thought to have mild anti-bacterial properties. Other bee products – royal jelly, propolis and bee pollen – are popularly taken as supplements for their purported health benefits.

Propolis

Bee propolis (or 'bee glue') is a sticky resin collected by bees from plants and trees; it has a strong, resinous smell, a bit like pine sap. Together with beeswax, it is used to build the beehive.

Although its healing properties have only been rediscovered in recent decades, its medicinal actions have been recorded since Greek and Roman times.

About half of bee propolis is resin, the rest is made up of wax, essential oils and pollen, plus trace amounts of vitamins, minerals and bioflavonoids (*see* Bioflavonoids, p. 56).

Propolis has been closely studied in Denmark, Eastern Europe, and in the USA, and so we have a good understanding of many of its actions.

Propolis has a strong antibiotic action, and may help our body's defences by neutralising foreign microbes. It also seems to have an antiviral and anti-fungal action. The active agents are as yet not fully known, but bioflavonoids are thought to be one of the key ingredients.

Traditionally, propolis has been used for healing cuts, sores, and wounds. Taken internally it may help combat colds, sore throats (gargle with it, too) and coughs. Other reported uses include helping to prevent peptic and duodenal ulcers, as propolis seems to fight Helicobacter pylori, the bacterium thought to be involved in some ulcer conditions.

Choosing A Propolis Supplement

Propolis capsules are found at around 500mg strengths. Take one daily for protective use, but you will need more (follow manufacturer's directions) if you want to help treat a minor condition.

Some concentrated propolis extracts are becoming available (equivalent to around 1000mg per capsule), but these may be chemically different from pure propolis.

Tinctures are available for internal or external use, e.g. as a gargle, mouthwash, antiseptic, or for sore gums and mouth ulcers.

Other Bee Products

Royal Jelly: This is a milky food produced by worker bees for the sustenance of their Queen. Royal jelly was once heralded by some as a 'miracle cure'. However, health claims concerning this substance have been largely unsubstantiated. It contains only trace amounts of certain vitamins and other nutrients.

Most people take royal jelly as a 'pick-me-up'; some claim that their hair, skin and nails improve with regular use of this supplement. Fresh royal jelly capsules are the most popular, and are usually available in strengths of 150mg–500mg. Less than 100mg – as in some combination products – is hardly worth having.

Freeze-dried, (or 'lyophilized') royal jelly capsules have the water removed, and are often cheaper to buy. You get a higher strength in one capsule, but proponents of 'fresh' royal jelly are adamant that the freeze-dried jelly is not as good. Such claims are hard to prove.

More concentrated liquid forms of royal jelly are also available.

Caution: In some countries, allergic reactions have very occasionally been reported in asthma sufferers taking royal jelly.

Bee Pollen: The pollen collected by bees may be formulated into granules or tablets. Some hayfever sufferers use bee pollen, as they report that it helps their symptoms when taken internally. However, allergic reactions may very occasionally result, so care must be taken. Tablets contain less bee pollen than granules, and are of very limited value nutritionally.

Kelp

Kelp is a general name applied to various seaweed species, commonly found on rocky coasts of Europe and North America.

What Does It Do?

The plant concentrates minerals from the sea and, if eaten as a food, can provide useful amounts of minerals. However, if taken as a food supplement, then the total daily amount of most nutrients will be small, with the exception of iodine.

Iodine is a trace element that forms a part of certain hormones (such as thyroxine) secreted by the thyroid gland. These hormones help to regulate the metabolic rate of the body, i.e. the rate at which we burn up our food. A lack of iodine in the diet may lead to the classic iodine deficiency disease, goitre, shown by a swelling of the thyroid gland in the neck. True iodine deficiency is rare in the UK.

Fish and other seafoods are the best common sources of iodine, though kelp is by far the richest source. Vegetables, cereals and most meats do contain very small quantities of iodine.

Iodine, in the form of kelp, is sometimes taken to stimulate a slightly underactive thyroid gland that does not require medical treatment (always see a doctor for diagnosis).

Choosing A Kelp Supplement

When comparing kelp products, the main points to look for are how much iodine you will get per daily dose (EC RDA = 150μg), and how many tablets you need to take daily. Most kelp products suggest at least three tablets daily, typically providing a total of 140μg–420μg iodine daily. Most good multivitamin formulations contain some iodine, too.

Some kelp products are fortified with a little extra calcium – check to see how much on the label. Kelp is sometimes also included in products aimed at slimmers, on the basis that the iodine content may help stimulate a sluggish metabolism. However, a calorie-controlled diet combined with exercise is the only true way to lose weight.

Safety

Avoid kelp during pregnancy, or if taking thyroxine. The maximum safe level of iodine from supplements (kelp and others) is thought to be 500μg a day.

Spirulina and Chlorella

These are two types of freshwater micro-algae, with broadly similar nutritional profiles. Both may be consumed as a powdered food or as tablets, but a typical supplemental intake

(3g a day) only provides nutritionally significant amounts of beta carotene, vitamin B12, iron and selenium. As a food (in amounts of around 20g) spirulina and chlorella provide significant amounts of a much wider range of nutrients, plus enzymes and other co-factors, and are a source of high-quality plant protein. In addition, spirulina can be a good provider of the important fatty acid GLA (100mg per 10g).

Spirulina, and especially chlorella, contain high concentrations of chlorophyll, the green plant pigment. At high levels, it is claimed that chlorophyll can help to remove heavy metals (lead, mercury, etc.) from the body, and to reduce the effects of radiation.

These 'green superfoods' are becoming more popular with vegans and vegetarians, but when used as a supplement, a lot of tablets need to be taken to obtain a beneficial level of nutrients. They may work out as an expensive way of getting supplemental nutrients.

CHAPTER FIVE

Common Questions on Supplements

Q. What is a 'food supplement'?

A. A food supplement is a tablet, capsule, powder or liquid providing vitamins, minerals or related dietary factors. Food supplements are meant to be taken in addition to your usual diet. They are not substitutes for proper food! Food supplements are legally classified as foods, and no medicinal claims can be made regarding their properties.

Q. Is it safe to take vitamin supplements during pregnancy?

A. With certain reservations, YES! The B vitamin folic acid has been proven to reduce the incidence of spina bifida and other birth defects and at least 400 microgrammes should be taken prior to conceiving and through the first three months of pregnancy. Calcium is another nutrient that is required in higher levels during pregnancy, and a supplement may be taken to boost levels. If you've always taken a multivitamin supplement prior to being pregnant, there's every reason for you to continue, providing the vitamin A content is low – government guidelines suggest a maximum of 800 microgrammes per day (unless in the form of beta carotene). Follow the guidelines in the sections on Safety: providing you don't breach these, your baby will be unharmed. With herbs, amino acids and other non-vitamin or mineral supplements, get your doctor's advice before you take them; evening primrose oil and fish oils are safe provided you only take the recommended amount on the label.

Q. What's the difference between a milligramme a microgramme and an international unit?

A. Most vitamins and minerals are only required in small milligramme (mg) quantities, with one milligramme being just one-thousandth (1/1000) of a gramme. Certain vitamins and trace minerals are needed in even tinier microgramme (µg) levels, where one microgramme equals 1/1000 of a miligramme or 1/1000000 (one millionth) of a gramme!

EC food labelling rules require that all vitamins and minerals be stated in weight terms – i.e. as mg or µg. However, many sources still refer to vitamins A, D and E in terms of international units (ius). International units measure the activity rather than the weight of the vitamin:

1 µg vitamin A = 3.33 iu

1 µg vitamin D = 40 iu

1 mg vitamin E = 1.49 iu

Q. I am taking a multivitamin, but I also want to make sure I am eating healthily. How can I improve my diet?

A. Eight simple guidelines for a healthy diet are:

1 Enjoy your food: healthy eating doesn't mean cutting out every food that tastes nice!

2 Eat a variety of different foods: the key to a balanced diet is consuming a wide range of foods, including bread, cereals and potatoes (starchy foods), fruit and vegetables, dairy foods (or calcium-rich alternatives) and meat/fish (or protein-rich alternatives).

3 Be a healthy weight: an underweight person may not eat enough essential nutrients, whilst an overweight person is

more likely to develop heart disease, diabetes and joint problems.

4   Eat plenty of foods rich in fibre: wholemeal bread, rice, pasta, cereals and potatoes supply fibre which prevents constipation and reduces the risk of common disorders of the intestine. Oats, beans, peas, lentils and fruit and vegetables supply soluble fibre which can help reduce the amount of cholesterol in the blood.

5   Don't eat too much fat: trim fat off meat, grill rather than fry, eat fish or poultry rather than red meat, and use fat-reduced dairy products. Look out for hidden fats in biscuits, cakes, etc.

6   Don't eat sugary foods too often: they cause tooth decay and aren't otherwise rich in nutrients.

7   Look after the vitamins and minerals in food: eat fresh fruit and vegetables as soon as possible after purchase, don't leave them soaking in water, and cook for the minimum amount of time, saving the cooking water for soups, gravies or sauces. Don't keep food hot for too long.

8   Keep alcohol within sensible limits: no more than 14 units a week for women and 21 units a week for men. (One unit equals half a pint of beer/lager, or one glass of wine, or one pub measure of spirits.)

These healthy-eating guidelines are suggested by the Ministry of Agriculture Fisheries and Food, and will help to ensure that you are getting a good basic diet. However, at times we do not eat well, or have extra nutrient needs – and this is where supplementation may be helpful.

Q. Is it safe to take supplements long-term?

A. As long as your daily nutrient intakes are within safe limits (*see* Vitamin and Mineral Safety, page 19), there is no reason why you should not carry on taking food supplements long term. However, always follow the pack directions carefully, and do not exceed the stated level of intake.

Q. What is the best time of day to take my supplements?

A. It doesn't matter what time of day you take your supplements, but taking them at the same time every day helps you to establish a routine. In the absence of any contrary information, always take supplements at meal-times (not on an empty stomach), since they function in combination with nutrients in food. Supplements should also be taken with a full glass of liquid for the best absorption. However, as always, follow the manufacturer's directions.

Q. How soon will I feel the benefits of taking a supplement?

A. If you start taking supplements as 'nutritional health insurance', don't suddenly expect to feel markedly different. Supplements will help make good any possible deficiencies in the diet, and may be helping to protect you against certain diseases in the long term.

If you are taking a supplement for a specific health benefit, then allow at least a month, and usually up to three months, before you make any judgements about its effect. Remember that strengths and dosages will affect results, and steps should also be taken to improve your diet.

Q. Are there any vitamins that might clash with others?

A. On the whole, no. Our bodies are designed to cope with digesting and absorbing the full range of vitamins, minerals, essential fatty acids, etc. at the same time – as, for example, when we eat a full meal. Excessive amounts of some nutrients, particularly minerals, may inhibit the absorption of others, but when supplements are used sensibly, and within safe limits, these interactions are, in practice, very rare (*see* Vitamin and Mineral Safety, p. 19).

Q. How can I be assured of the quality of supplements?

A. Food law exists to ensure the safety and quality of food and food supplements, but buying a reputable brand is always good advice. The Council for Responsible Nutrition – representing the vast majority of supplement sales in the UK – has issued specific Good Manufacturing Guidelines for food supplements which many companies have undertaken to follow. These guidelines establish very high standards for quality and purity of supplements.

Q. How should I store my supplements?

A. You should store your supplements in a cool, dry place that is away from direct heat and light. Keep supplements, especially those containing iron – which can be dangerous at excessive levels – out of children's reach, and close the cap tightly.

Q. Is the 'best before' date important on supplements?

A. The 'best before' date on the label indicates the date up to which the full potency of the product can be guaranteed (providing the supplement is stored as directed). Whilst the potency may decline, the safety of the product is not usually at risk after this time.

INDEX